Aktuelle Forschung Medizintechnik

Editor-in-Chief:
Th. M. Buzug, Lübeck, Deutschland

Unter den Zukunftstechnologien mit hohem Innovationspotenzial ist die Medizintechnik in Wissenschaft und Wirtschaft hervorragend aufgestellt, erzielt überdurchschnittliche Wachstumsraten und gilt als krisensichere Branche. Wesentliche Trends der Medizintechnik sind die Computerisierung, Miniaturisierung und Molekularisierung. Die Computerisierung stellt beispielsweise die Grundlage für die medizinische Bildgebung, Bildverarbeitung und bildgeführte Chirurgie dar. Die Miniaturisierung spielt bei intelligenten Implantaten, der minimalinvasiven Chirurgie, aber auch bei der Entwicklung von neuen nanostrukturierten Materialien eine wichtige Rolle in der Medizin. Die Molekularisierung ist unter anderem in der regenerativen Medizin, aber auch im Rahmen der sogenannten molekularen Bildgebung ein entscheidender Aspekt. Disziplinen übergreifend sind daher Querschnittstechnologien wie die Nano- und Mikrosystemtechnik, optische Technologien und Softwaresysteme von großem Interesse.

Diese Schriftenreihe für herausragende Dissertationen und Habilitationsschriften aus dem Themengebiet Medizintechnik spannt den Bogen vom Klinikingenieurwesen und der Medizinischen Informatik bis hin zur Medizinischen Physik, Biomedizintechnik und Medizinischen Ingenieurwissenschaft.

Alexander Schmidt-Richberg

Registration Methods for Pulmonary Image Analysis

Integration of Morphological
and Physiological Knowledge

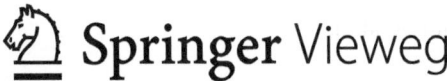 Springer Vieweg

Alexander Schmidt-Richberg
University of Lübeck
Germany

Dissertation University of Lübeck, 2013

ISBN 978-3-658-01661-6   ISBN 978-3-658-01662-3 (eBook)
DOI 10.1007/978-3-658-01662-3

The Deutsche Nationalbibliothek lists this publication in the Deutsche Nationalbibliografie; detailed bibliographic data are available in the Internet at http://dnb.d-nb.de.

Library of Congress Control Number: 2014931204

Springer Vieweg
© Springer Fachmedien Wiesbaden 2014

Printed on acid-free paper

Springer Vieweg is a brand of Springer DE.
Springer DE is part of Springer Science+Business Media.
www.springer-vieweg.de

Preface by the Series Editor

The book "Registration Methods for Pulmonary Image Analysis. Integration of Morphological and Physiological Knowledge" by Dr. Alexander Schmidt-Richberg is the seventh volume of the new Springer-Vieweg series of excellent theses in medical engineering. The thesis of Dr. Schmidt-Richberg has been selected by an editorial board of highly recognized scientists working in that field.

The Springer-Vieweg series aims to establish a forum for Monographs and Proceedings on Medical Engineering. The series publishes works that give insights into the novel developments in that field. Prospective authors may contact the Series Editor about future publications within the series at:

Prof. Dr. Thorsten M. Buzug
Series Editor Medical Engineering

Institute of Medical Engineering
University of Lübeck
Ratzeburger Allee 160
23562 Lübeck

Web: www.imt.uni-luebeck.de
Email: buzug@imt.uni-luebeck.de

Foreword

Medical image registration and segmentation of 3D and 4D image data are challenging problems in the field of medical image computing. In this book, Alexander Schmidt-Richberg focuses on the integrated registration and segmentation of the lung and lung lobes in 3D and 4D CT image data. While 3D images reflect the spatial structure and relationship of organs and pathological structures, spatio-temporal image data sets – so called 4D image data – enable the analysis of the dynamic behavior of organs and tumors, e.g. during breathing. The presented image processing techniques allow the extraction of additional information from 3D and 4D images in a new quality. While the segmentation of image data is the basis for the quantitative analysis and 3D visualization of organs and pathologies, with image registration methods an alignment of image data becomes possible so that corresponding image structures are assigned to each other. Hence, breathing induced motion as well as morphological changes of organs and tumors can be analyzed by the registration of CT scans of one patient generated at different time points. This is important for the monitoring of disease progression and ventilation assessment as well as in the context of radiotherapy, where the registration of 4D CT images is used to analyze breathing motion.

In this book, Alexander Schmidt-Richberg presents new integrated registration and segmentation techniques for pulmonary image analysis. He develops two approaches in which segmentations of specific structures are employed to integrate anatomical and physiological knowledge into the registration algorithm. On the one hand, the sliding motion at the lung boundaries is modeled directly in the registration approach. This specific characteristic of lung physiology plays an important role, because the discontinuous nature of the sliding lung motion cannot be described accurately using common non-linear registration methods. On the other hand, a segmentation of the pulmonary lobes is integrated into the registration method to align the interlobular fissures. Lung lobe registration is challenging due to the extremely low contrast in CT images, which results in unsatisfying results with conventional approaches. The presented approach enables an alignment of the lung lobes by considering the morphological knowledge about the lung provided by integrated segmentations. With the combined segmentation and registration approach he shows that an explicit consideration of morphological and physiological a priori knowledge about the lung can considerably improve registration accuracy and plausibility.

This book provides the reader with a deep insight into the field of image registration and segmentation including a thorough introduction to the mathematical background. Moreover, the problem-specific adaption of registration approaches is demonstrated. Many medical examples illustrate the methods and give the reader an impression of the application of the methods in practice. This book is highly recommended for all readers interested in the registration and segmentation of medical image data.

Lübeck, December 2013

Prof. Dr. rer. nat. habil. Heinz Handels
Institute of Medical Informatics
University of Lübeck

Acknowledgments

A research project like this is never the work of one person alone. I was fortunate enough to find a not only very productive but also warm and friendly environment to work on my thesis. I would therefore like to thank all the people who contributed in one way or the other to the work described in this manuscript.

I thank my doctoral advisor Prof. Dr. Heinz Handels for his support and for providing a welcoming and warm atmosphere at the Institute of Medical Informatics of the University Hospital Center Hamburg-Eppendorf and later at the University of Lübeck. He has always been very encouraging and inspiring and admitted me enough freedom to concentrate on the thesis. Furthermore, I'd like to thank my co-referee Prof. Dr. Thorsten Buzug and Prof. Dr. Alfred Mertins for chairing.

My very special thanks go to Jan Ehrhardt and René Werner. We have not only worked very closely together but have also become close friends over the past years. Jan has introduced me to the world of medical imaging and guided me all the way through my Diploma and PhD thesis, providing many essential inspirations. René has always been incredibly supportive and a role model in many ways. I also thank my colleagues and dear friends Heike Hufnagel and Nils Forkert for providing input for and – at least equally important – distraction from my work. Thank you, Jan, René, Heike and Nils. You have been the best team anyone could hope for and I will always miss our coffee breaks.

I further thank my colleagues at the IMIs in Lübeck and Hamburg, with whom I had a great time: André, Anni, Dennis, Dirk, Gabi, Jan-Hinrich, Josef, Jule, Kerstin, Martin, Matthias Färber, Matthias Wilms (particularly for enduring my endless chatting in our office) and Mirko. Moreover, I thank Susanne and Renate for saving me from my chaotic organisation on several occasions. I would like to thank Xavier Pennec for my time in France and for letting me witness his phenomenal fascination for digging deep into the mathematical foundations. Working with him has been an inspiration.

I am very grateful for the funding sources that allowed me to pursue my research: the German Research Foundation (DFG) and the German Academic Exchange Service (DAAD).

Finally, with all my heart I thank my parents Monika and Dieter as well as my sister Stefanie with her family. It is an immense help that I can always trust in their love, belief and support of every possible kind. I thank all my dear friends who let me enjoy every day of my doctorate: Only a happy PhD student is a good PhD student! I also deeply thank Alena for the wonderful time we shared.

Abstract

In this thesis, methods for the registration of pulmonary CT images are developed in which segmentations are used to model lung-specific morphological and physiological aspects of the lung.

Various applications in the field of pulmonary image analysis require a registration of CT images of the lung. It is needed, for example, to align different scans of one patient for assessing local ventilation parameters or monitoring disease progression. A registration-based estimation of the breathing motion is employed to increase accuracy in radiotherapy. Moreover, the registration of scans of different patients is required for atlas-based segmentation and motion modeling. While several different registration techniques have been developed in the past, the image content is often regarded as a homogeneous structure and no specific characteristics of the lung are modeled. In this work, the hypothesis is followed that an explicit consideration of morphological and physiological aspects of the lung can considerably improve registration accuracy and plausibility. For this purpose, two approaches are developed in which segmentations of specific organs are employed to integrate such knowledge into the registration algorithm. In the first part, a method for integrated segmentation and registration is presented to explicitly align the pulmonary lobes. It is motivated by the observation that conventional intensity-based registration approaches often expose an insufficient lobe alignment because the interlobular fissures are very low-contrasted in CT images and therefore provide little information for the algorithm. This problem is addressed in two steps: First, an automatic approach for lobe segmentation is presented in which shape information is incorporated by a novel force term. The term relies on a supervised fissure detection and causes an attraction of the contour in direction of the lobe boundaries. Then, the segmentation component is integrated into the registration framework. In this way, an alignment of the fissures is explicitly promoted.

In the second part, a segmentation is used to model physiological properties of the breathing motion at the lung boundaries. In this region, respiration causes inner and outer lung pleura to slide along each other, which entails discontinuities in the motion field. Such sliding motion contradicts the smoothing employed in most registration algorithms and entails severe errors in the estimation if not properly accounted for. To remedy this problem, a new segmentation-based regularization approach is presented in which normal- and tangential-directed motion are regarded separately. This allows a physiologically plausible modeling of the sliding motion at the lung boundaries.

Both approaches are extensively evaluated using clinical CT images, including publicly available data to allow a comparison with other approaches. The evaluation shows that improvements over state-of-the-art techniques can be obtained using the developed methods. It is concluded that a segmentation-based consideration of lung morphology and physiology is beneficial for registration accuracy and plausibility.

Contents

Chapter 1

Introduction

The analysis of pulmonary images is of eminent importance in modern medicine. Computed tomography (CT) scans of the thorax, for example, enable a three-dimensional insight into the patient's anatomy and are used to non-invasively study morphology and function of the lung with application to diagnosis, treatment and monitoring of various pulmonary diseases. In this context, the role of techniques for computer-aided image analysis is manyfold. For example, they are used to extract quantitative values about the type and growth of pulmonary nodules to early diagnose malignant neoplasms of lung and bronchus [Armato and Sensakovic 2004], which are responsible for the most cancer-related deaths in the US [ACS 2011]. After diagnosis, lung CT scans are used to plan and guide interventions or radiotherapy and to monitor success of the treatment [Yan et al. 1999]. Functional pulmonary image analysis is further used for a regional assessment of ventilation and perfusion parameters to quantify gas exchange [Hoffman et al. 2004], which is of interest for the diagnosis of fibrosis or Chronic Obstructive Pulmonary Diseases (COPD) such as emphysema [Scatarige et al. 2003].

For many of those applications, it is necessary to establish correspondences between anatomical points and structures contained in two or more CT scans. This is a non-trivial task since the images might be acquired at different points of time, with different devices, or of different subjects. Consequently, patients are often positioned differently in the scanner and they are subject to internal motion and daily variations of the morphology. To tackle this problem, several computer-based methods have been developed that aim at mapping points or structures from one image to the corresponding points of another image. This procedure is called *image registration*.

The use of registration techniques for pulmonary image analysis is diverse. On the one hand, it is often necessary to conflate the information contained in two or more scans, a process also called image fusion. Referring to the applications mentioned above, a fusion-based alignment of longitudinal CT scans is for example utilized to monitor progression of diseases as nodules [Zheng et al. 2007; Staring et al. 2009] or emphysema [Gorbunova et al. 2010]. In other scenarios, the generation of a normative atlas of the lung is in the focus, which allows performing statistics on physiological aspects and determining, for example, the normal range of intensity variations [Li et al. 2012]. For this task,

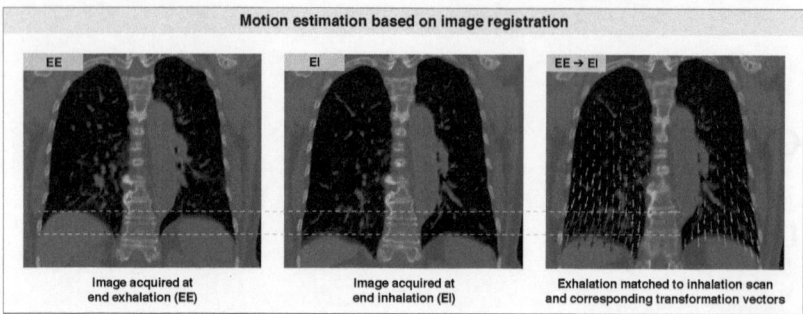

Figure 1.1: CT images of the lung acquired during end exhalation (EE, left) and end inhalation (EI, center). By a registration of the images, the exhale scan can be matched to the inhale scan, such that anatomically corresponding points have the same coordinates. The resulting transformation (right) then describes the breathing-induced lung motion. The horizontal lines highlight the motion of the diaphragm.

inter-patient registration is employed to map a set of images of different subjects to a common coordinate system and thereby establish correspondences between the patients [Ehrhardt et al. 2011]. The same technique is needed for atlas-based segmentation, which are also of high clinical relevance. Here, to outline anatomical objects like the lungs or the pulmonary lobes, annotated reference data sets are propagated to a new subject. In this way, conclusions on shape and position of organs in the patient image can be drawn [van Rikxoort et al. 2010].

Apart from image fusion, another major field of application for registration algorithms is the estimation of motion: If two CT scans of a patient acquired at end inhalation and end exhalation are registered, the obtained transformation specifies the breathing-induced motion of each tissue point (see Figure 1.1). This information can be used, for example, to quantify lung ventilation by either looking at the change of intensity between corresponding voxels [Castillo et al. 2010b] or assessing the local volume change directly from the deformation [Reinhardt et al. 2008].

Recent developments in CT imaging allow to go even one step further because with time-resolved 4D CT scans it became possible to image the lung during the whole breathing cycle and thereby further study pulmonary kinetics [Tustison et al. 2011]. A registration of the temporal frames of a 4D data set yields trajectories describing the breathing-induced motion of each tissue point during the respiratory cycle (see Figure 1.2). This is essential for radiation therapy of lung tumors to increase the accuracy of dose delivery [Yan et al. 1999; Sarrut 2006].

As these examples demonstrate, the scope of registration techniques in pulmonary image analysis is diverse. In the following, registration-based 4D risk assessment for radiotherapy is exemplarily detailed to illustrate the integration of registration algorithms into the clinical workflow.

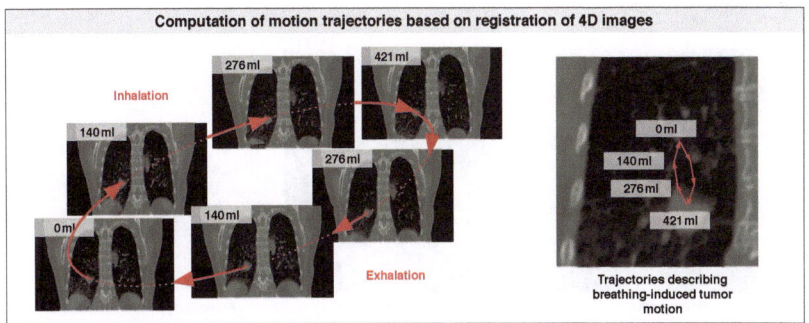

Figure 1.2: By registration of the frames of a time-resolved 4D CT set, the concatenation of the transformation vectors describes the path of each tissue point during the breathing cycle. In this figure, the numbers indicate the respective lung volume. It is to be noted that the path during inhalation usually diverges from the path during exhalation, which is known as hysteresis.

1.1 Registration in pulmonary image analysis: 4D risk assessment for radiotherapy as an example

Respiratory motion is a major challenge in radiation therapy of lung tumors, which is intended to deliver a desired dose to the target volume while limiting radiation of surrounding healthy tissues. Moving targets, however, cause an uncertainty of the exact tumor location during therapy. In conventional therapy, this is accounted for during treatment planning by the definition of large safety margins around the tumor and delivering a dose to the whole region [ICRU 1999, 2010]. Obviously, this technique contradicts the aim of limiting damage to healthy tissue.

With the invention of 4D CT imaging, assessing information about the patient-specific respiratory motion became possible. This led to the development of several techniques to address moving targets in radiotherapy [Keall et al. 2006]. For example, in 4D treatment planning, precise knowledge about lung and tumor motion is used to optimize the treatment plan by appropriately dimensioning safety margins [Ezhil et al. 2008]. In respiratory gating methods [Mageras and Yorke 2004] and advanced techniques like real-time tumor tracking [Shimizu et al. 2001], tumor motion is correlated with the motion of internal or external markers in or on a patient, respectively. These markers are then tracked during therapy and used to either trigger dose application at a certain breathing state (gating) or move the radiation source depending on the actual position of the target volume. More facile to integrate in the clinical routine is a 4D risk assessment, in which the influence of breathing motion on dose application is estimated and evaluated [Yan et al. 1999; Werner et al. 2012a]. For this purpose, a conventional 3D treatment plan is generated based on a reference time point of a 4D

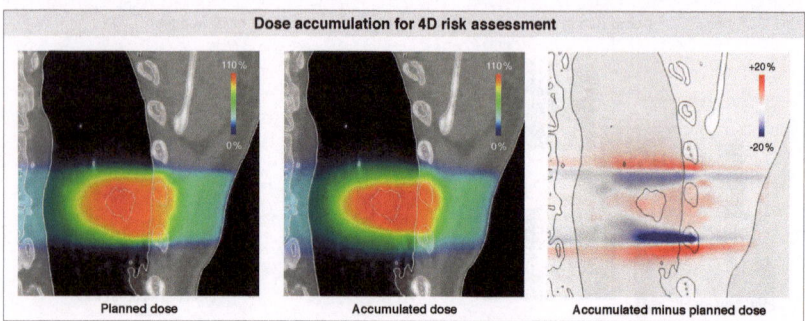

Figure 1.3: Comparison of the planned dose using a static 3D CT scan (left) and the accumulated dose computed based on a 4D CT sequence using image registration techniques (center). The color overlay signifies the applied dose with 100% being the prescribed dose. The influence of breathing motion on the dose distribution is visible in particular in the difference image (right). Blue and red regions indicate an under- and overdosage, respectively. Illustration following [Werner et al. 2012a].

CT sequence, that means a static 3D CT scan. In the next step, registration methods are applied on the whole image sequence to estimate the patient-specific deformation of the lung during the breathing cycle, as illustrated in Figure 1.2. For each tissue point, this information is then used to simulate the effectively delivered dose depending on its actual position during the treatment. This procedure is called dose accumulation. Finally, the accumulated dose is compared to the initially planned dose and validated by a clinical expert to ensure that a breathing-induced underdosage of the target volume is avoided and damage to healthy tissue and organs-at-risk is within an acceptable range (see Figure 1.3).

This example shows that motion estimation of the lung based on 4D image data is of high clinical relevance. In a task group report on radiation oncology by the American Association of Physicists in Medicine (AAPM), the necessity of developing *"robust deformable image-registration algorithms to facilitate dose accumulation due to anatomy deformation"* is therefore underlined [Keall et al. 2006].

In clinical practice, the problem arises that 4D CT imaging is currently not the standard procedure in many institutions, which is obstructive for the employment of 4D risk assessment (as well as for other approaches for motion compensation). However, human breathing patterns are very similar between the patients: While the largest motion amplitudes arise close to the diaphragm, the tip of the lung barely moves. Based on these observations, Ehrhardt et al. [2011] aimed to generate a model that describes the mean human breathing motion and to apply this model to approximate the specific motion of a patient without any 4D image data available. First, results presented by Werner et al. [2012b] suggest that – under certain conditions to tumor size and location – the mean model provides valuable information about the patient's breathing physiology when applied to estimate dose distribution.

Several registration-based steps are required to generate the mean motion model based on a set of 4D CT scans. First, patient-specific motion fields are computed for each subject of the pool. To relate these individual estimates, a mean shape and intensity atlas of the lung is computed from all data sets. Subsequently, all motion fields are transferred to the coordinate system of the atlas and then averaged. Furthermore, for the application of the atlas to a 3D scan of a specific patient, this image is then registered with the intensity atlas and the mean motion is transferred accordingly.[1]

Modeling mean patient motion demonstrates an additional utilization of registration algorithms, which are not only required for the patient-specific motion estimation, but also to establish plausible correspondences between different patients. Such an inter-patient registration raises further requirements on the algorithm because differences between the morphologies have to be overcome.

1.2 Objectives

The given examples demonstrate that precise algorithms for lung registration are of high relevance for radiotherapy and – as initially detailed – in the much larger scope of pulmonary image analysis. Various generic registration approaches have been proposed in the past and applied to thoracic CT images. However, the image is usually regarded as a homogeneous structure and no specific characteristics of the lung are modeled.

The purpose of this work is therefore to take advantage of the morphological knowledge provided by a segmentation to improve registration algorithms. With this aim in mind, two main aspects are regarded. On the one hand, segmentations supply information about the anatomy that can be directly used to align certain structures. On the other hand, the information can be used to model physiological properties of the lung motion. As the following examples demonstrate, both aspects are of relevance for pulmonary image registration, because they tackle limitations of common, solely intensity-based approaches.

Alignment of pulmonary lobes   The human lungs consist of five individual lobes, two in the left and three in the right lung. Adhering lobes are divided by double layers of visceral pleurae, called the interlobular fissures. However, fissures are barely visible in CT scans, which often leads to an insufficient alignment of the lobes by registration algorithms and consequently incorrectly established correspondences. Due to variances

---

[1]   Technically, to generate the mean motion model and to adapt it to a patient anatomy, a further parameter is required to account for different depths of breathing. This is not further discussed at this point. For details, the reader is referred to [Ehrhardt et al. 2011].

in the patients' anatomies, this is especially severe for the registration of different subjects, but the problem also arises for motion estimation based on images of a single patient.

Sliding motion at lung boundaries   Registration algorithms generally incorporate some kind of smoothing – also called regularization – to ensure physiologically plausible transformations. However, at the lung boundaries, inner and outer pleura of the lung slide along each other causing discontinuities in the motion field. This contradicts a globally homogeneous regularization and entails severe errors in the estimated motion field if not properly accounted for.

Motivated by these observations, new approaches are to be developed in this work to optimize registration algorithms specifically for the human lungs. This aim is followed by incorporation segmentations of the relevant structures (lung or pulmonary lobes) in the model to integrate knowledge about the patient's morphology. Moreover, the developed methods are to be thoroughly evaluated on the base of clinical image data to demonstrate their applicability.

1.3 Structure of this thesis

Pursuing the presented objectives, this work is organized as follows:

In **Chapter 2**, an overview on current methods for lung registration is given. The focus is on the four main components of registration algorithms: similarity measure, transformation model, regularization and solution strategy.

In **Chapters 3 and 4**, the mathematical foundations of image registration and level set-based segmentation are detailed. Both methods are formulated as modular variational frameworks, which allow an application-specific adaption of the algorithms and an intrinsic combination of registration and segmentation. Synthetic examples are given to demonstrate the functionality of the individual modules based on synthetic image data.

In **Chapters 5 and 6**, models for novel registration approaches are derived. On the one hand, an integrated registration and segmentation method is presented to explicitly align the pulmonary lobes. For this purpose, a new approach for level set-based segmentation of the pulmonary lobes is proposed and then incorporated in the registration framework. On the other hand, a segmentation-based method for direction-dependent regularization is presented with the aim of preserving sliding motion at the lung boundaries. As in the preceding chapters, the functionality of the algorithms is illustrated using synthetic images.

In **Chapter 7**, an extensive evaluation study is provided based on clinical CT scans. Following a presentation of the utilized image data, an overview on the metrics used for quantitative quality assessment of registration and segmentation algorithms is given. Afterwards, the registration framework introduced in Chapter 3 is optimized with respect to various tasks of pulmonary image analysis, which are in detail motion estimation, general intra-patient registration and inter-patient registration for atlas generation. In the subsequent sections, the proposed methods for lobe segmentation, registration with fissure alignment and direction-dependent regularization are profoundly tested.

In **Chapter 8**, a discussion of the developed methods is provided. In particular, strengths and limitations are summarized, clinical relevance and applicability are assessed, and an outlook on further developments is given.

1.4 Publications

Parts of this work have been published before in journal articles or conference proceedings. The application-specific optimization of the basic registration framework is described in [Schmidt-Richberg et al. 2010a] and [Werner et al. 2009b] under significant participation of the author. The registration with explicit fissure alignment was developed in [Schmidt-Richberg et al. 2012c] (fissure detection), [Schmidt-Richberg et al. 2012d] (lobe segmentation), [Schmidt-Richberg et al. 2009c] (integrated framework) and [Schmidt-Richberg et al. 2012b] (final approach). The direction-dependent regularization for modeling sliding motion was first presented in [Schmidt-Richberg et al. 2009b] and extended to liver sliding in [Schmidt-Richberg et al. 2010b]. An alternative not relying on a lung segmentation was presented in [Schmidt-Richberg et al. 2012e]. Considerable improvements in the numerical solution were proposed in [Schmidt-Richberg et al. 2012a]. Further articles have been published under participation of the author in the context of respiratory motion modeling, dose accumulation, shape-based level set segmentation and vessel segmentation.

Chapter 2

Current methods for lung registration

The determination of correspondences between two or more images is required in almost every field of medical image processing. Consequently, a vast diversity of registration algorithms has been developed in the past, which is documented by several review articles [Brown 1992; Maintz and Viergever 1998; Hill et al. 2001; Zitova and Flusser 2003; Oliveira and Tavares 2012; Sotiras et al. 2012] and books [Hajnal et al. 2001; Modersitzki 2004; Goshtasby 2012a] published on this topic.

As initially detailed, an important field of application of registration techniques is the correspondence analysis in lung CT images. Focussing on this field, the domain of algorithms can be restricted to monomodal 3D-3D registration methods, but it still offers a variety of different approaches. To assess and compare their accuracy, the demand for common evaluation platforms has emerged in recent years. As a consequence, two international evaluation studies have been conducted in 2009 and 2010.

On the one hand, several academic and commercial institutions were invited to participate at the *Multi-Institution Deformable Registration Accuracy Study* (MIDRAS), with the purpose *"to assess the accuracy, reproducibility, and computational performance of deformable image registration algorithms under development at multiple institutions on common datasets."* [Brock et al. 2010]. Altogether, twenty-one groups submitted their results. In addition to thoracic 4D CT scans, CT and MR images of liver and prostate were considered in this study.

On the other hand, the *Evaluation of Methods for Pulmonary Image REgistration 2010* (EMPIRE10) challenge is an ongoing study and was initiated in conjunction with the MICCAI 2010 conference at Beijing, China [Murphy et al. 2011b]. Focussing on lung registration, it is aimed at registering 30 thoracic CT scan pairs covering different fields of intra-patient registration. Results are then evaluated with a common set of criteria. Here, initially twenty-three groups submitted thirty-four algorithms to compete in the challenge.

Moreover, with the publically available POPI model [Vandemeulebroucke et al. 2007] and the DIR-lab data [Castillo et al. 2009], several 4D CT scans have been provided together with manually determined corresponding points to enable the quantitative evaluation of registration algorithms for motion estimation. These images are referred to in many recent publications dealing with lung registration to provide a more meaningful comparison. For more details on POPI, DIR-lab and the EMPIRE challenge, the reader is referred to Sections 7.1.2 and 7.2.3.

In this chapter, an overview on current methods for the registration of thoracic CT images is given. Since collating a comprehensive survey on lung registration techniques would surpass the scope of this work, the focus is on methods participating in one of the aforementioned challenges as well as very recent developments in this field. These algorithms are listed in Table 2.1. In Section 2.1, the approaches are categorized and different possibilities for the definition of their fundamental components highlighted.[1] Available open-source implementations are introduced in Section 2.2 and the implications on this thesis derived in Section 2.3.

2.1 Intensity-based registration techniques

Let T and R denote two images (for example, two time points of a 4D sequence), called template and reference image. The goal of image registration is finding a transformation φ that warps a template image to match a reference image, such that $T \circ \varphi \approx R$. A commonly persuaded approach to find φ is by minimization of an energy functional

$$\mathcal{J}[\varphi] := \mathcal{D}[T \circ \varphi, R],$$

where $\mathcal{D}$ is a distance measure that quantifies the dissimilarity between reference and transformed template image. In this formulation, two components have to be determined: the distance measure to precisely define the sense of similarity and the transformation model. However, depending on the degrees of freedom of the transformation, an additional condition is often required to restrain it to be physiologically plausible. Since the lung can be described as an elastic body [Tustison et al. 2011], a certain smoothness of the transformation is expected and can be achieved by adding a regularization condition $\mathcal{S}$ to the energy functional:

$$\mathcal{J}[\varphi] := \mathcal{D}[T \circ \varphi, R] + \mathcal{S}[\varphi]. \tag{2.1}$$

In the following Sections 2.1.1 to 2.1.3, an overview on different transformation models, regularizers and distance measures that are currently used in the literature is given. From a computational point of view, the optimization strategy for finding the minimum of the functional is also of eminent importance. Different approaches for this purpose are described in Section 2.1.4.

---

[1] Since the focus is on the evaluation studies, this overview is restrained to intensity-based approaches. Shape- and feature-based registration methods – usually used in a pre-processing step to overcome anatomical differences and divergences in patient positioning, especially in inter-subject registration – are not further regarded at this point.

Table 2.1: Current methods for lung CT registration. The ten best-ranked methods of the MIDRAS [Brock et al. 2010] and EMPIRE10 [Murphy et al. 2011b] studies are compared. Furthermore, some recent methods are listed that follow noteworthy ideas. **Abbreviations:** TPS: Thin-plate-splines; (N)MI: (Normalized) Mutual Information; SAD: Sum of Absolute Difference; (N)SSD: (Normalized) Sum of Squared Differences; NCC: Normalized Cross Correlation; SSTVD: Sum of Squared Tissue Volume Differences; SSVMD: Sum of Squared Vesselness Measure Differences; NGF: Normalized Gradient Field; ELE: Euler-Lagrange Equation; GD: Gradient Descent; CG: Conjugated Gradients; ASGD: Adaptive Stochastic Gradient Descent; BFGS: Broyden-Fletcher-Goldfarb-Shanno; MRF: Markov Random Fields; **References:** M1: Dong, Zhang [Wang et al. 2005]; M2: Han; M3: Dufort, Stundiza; M4: Xia, Samant; M5: El Naqa, Yang [Yang et al. 2008]; M6: Hawkes, Crum [Crum et al. 2005]; M7: Heath [Heath et al. 2007]; M8: Mageras, Hu [Lu et al. 2004]; M9: Nord; M10: Noe, Tanderup [Noe et al. 2008]; E1: [Han 2010]; E2: [Song et al. 2010]; E3: [Staring et al. 2010]; E4: [Schmidt-Richberg et al. 2010a]; E5: [Modat et al. 2010a]; E6: [Kabus and Lorenz 2010]; E7: [Cao et al. 2010b]; E8: [Muenzing et al. 2010]; E9: [Song et al. 2010]; E10: [Garcia et al. 2010]; F1: [Heinrich et al. 2012]; F2: [Rühaak et al. 2013]; F3: [Gorbunova et al. 2012]

Ref.	Transform. model	Regularizer	Distance measure	Solver
\- MIDRAS STUDY \-				
M1	Dense field	Gaussian	NSSD	Demons-like
M2	B-splines	not specified	SSD	GD
M3	TPS	Bending energy	SSD	Backward GD
M4	Dense field	Diffusion-based	SSD	GD
M5	Dense field	Gaussian	MSD	Gauss-Seidel
M6	Dense field	Viscous-fluid	NCC	Full Multigrid
M7	Dense field	Linear-elastic	NCC	3D Simplex
M8	Dense field	Diffusion	SSD	ELE/Gauss-Seidel
M9	Dense field	Gaussian	NSSD	Demons-like
M10	Dense field	Viscous-fluid	SSD	GD
\- EMPIRE10 STUDY \-				
E1	Dense field	Gaussian	MI/NSSD*	pair-and-smooth
E2	Diffeomorphic	Gaussian	NCC	ELE/GD
E3	B-splines	not specified	NCC	ASGD
E4	Diffeomorphic	Diffusion	NSSD	ELE/GD
E5	B-splines	Bending energy	NMI	CG
E6	Dense field	Linear-elastic	SSD	ELE/GD
E7	B-splines	Laplacian	SSTVD/SSVMD	Quasi-Newton (BFGS)
E8	Diffeomorphic	Diffusion	NSSD	Demons-like
E9	Diffeomorphic	Gaussian	NCC	ELE/GD
E10	Diffeomorphic	Gaussian	NSSD	Demons-like
\- FURTHER APPROACHES \-				
F1	Diffeomorphic	Total variation	SAD	MRF on spanning tree
F2	Dense field	Curvature	NGF	L-BFGS
F3	B-splines	not specified	Mass-preserving	ASGD

* In this approach, additional features are detected and incorporated in the registration.

2.1.1 Transformation models

Affine transformations   Affine or rigid body transformations are frequently used for the alignment of brain images. Due to the very low number of parameters that have to be determined, linear registration is usually very performant. However, the complex deformation of an elastic organ like the lung cannot be described appropriately by such a simplistic transformation model. Therefore, affine transformations are rarely applied for lung registration aside from a pre-alignment. The same holds true for piecewise affine or poly-affine transformations [Arsigny et al. 2006b].

Spline-based transformations   Spline-based transformation models are inspired by interpolation theory. The transformation is explicitly given for a set of control points and interpolated for the rest of the domain. In early approaches, radial basis functions like thin-plate-splines (TPS) [Bookstein 1989] or physically motivated elastic-body-splines [Davis et al. 1997] were applied. Free-form deformations (FFD) also gained a wide acceptance in image registration [Rueckert et al. 1999]. Here, locally controlled B-splines are used to interpolate between the control points of a rectangular grid, which entails computational benefits. In gerneral, spline-based transformations unite a high flexibility with a (compared to dense transformations) relatively low number of parameters.

Dense displacement fields   Since Thirion [1995] presented the demons-based registration, transformations are often defined by a dense vector field in which the vector attached to each voxel describes the displacement of the corresponding point. This approach is followed by 17 of the 23 methods listed in Table 2.1. Dense transformations entail increased demands on the computational resources but represent the most flexible deformation model. Due to this, they have to be employed in connection with a suitable regularizer that ensures physiologically plausible transformations.

Diffeomorphic transformations   Following the argumentation of Beg et al. [2005], constraining the transformation to be a diffeomorphism is a natural choice in medical image registration as "connected sets remain connected, disjoint sets remain disjoint [and] the smoothness of anatomical features [...] is preserved." From a mathematical perspective, this can be achieved by imposing additional requirements on the displacement field. For example, in the *Large Deformation Diffeomorphic Metric Mapping* (LDDMM) framework presented by Beg et al. [2005], diffeomorphic transformations are parameterized as the flow over a time-dependent velocity field. Arsigny et al. [2006a] proposed to use stationary velocity fields instead, which considerably increases computational efficiency at the expense of flexibility. Other approaches exist that guarantee, for example, diffeomorphic free-form deformations [Rueckert et al. 2006].

2.1.2 Regularization approaches

The regularization approach is closely related to the transformation model and applied to restrict the domain of valid deformations. Focussing on the regularization of dense displacement fields, the most common approaches are summarized in the following.

Gaussian/Diffusion Thirion [1995] first applied a component-wise Gaussian smoothing of the displacement field. As derived in [Modersitzki 2004], this is closely related to a diffusion regularization, in which large gradients in the field are penalized for each component independently. Both approaches can be computed very efficiently and are therefore frequently used in current registration approaches (see Table 2.1). However, they lack a physical motivation.

Elastic body In this approach, the image domain is modeled as an elastic body based on the Navier-Cauchy equation [Broit 1981]. The Lamé parameters μ and λ are used to influence the material properties. Various extensions have been proposed that tackle problems like inverse consistency [Christensen and Johnson 2001], large deformations [Pennec et al. 2005] and numerical efficiency [Fischer and Modersitzki 1999].

Viscous flow Christensen et al. [1996] first introduced viscous flow transformations into image registration. Based on the Navier-Stokes equation, the image domain is modeled as a viscous fluid. Since not the deformation but the underlying velocity field is regularized, this approach allows large deformations. However, computational inefficiency is a fundamental drawback of this model and consequently most developments concentrate on improving the numerical performance, for example based on scale-space filtering [Bro-Nielsen and Gramkow 1996] or multigrid techniques [Crum et al. 2005].

Curvature Curvature regularization was introduced by Fischer and Modersitzki [2004] and defined to penalize the Laplacian of the displacement field, which is an approximation of its curvature. The major advantage of this approach is that affine transformations are not penalized. Therefore, misalignments can be accounted for without an additional pre-registration step. In [Beuthien et al. 2010], curvature regularization is efficiently solved by recursive filtering based on the Green's function.

Total variation Regularization based on the total variation or the L_1 norm of the displacement field was employed for image registration in [Frohn-Schauf et al. 2007]. Since it is more robust to outliers than the diffusion approach, it is mainly used to model discontinuous motion in computer vision. However, total variation has also been applied to lung CT registration [Heinrich et al. 2012].

2.1.3 Distance measures

A comprehensive overview on distance and similarity metrics if given in [Goshtasby 2012b] and – focussing on multimodal registration – in [Hermosillo et al. 2002]. Here, only approaches frequently applied to lung registration are outlined.

Sum of Squared Differences Most intuitively, image similarity is measured by regarding the intensity differences in each voxel, which leads to the definition of the Sum of Absolute or Squared Differences (SAD and SSD) as distance measures. SSD can be shown to be the optimal measure when two images only differ by Gaussian noise [Hill et al. 2001], which leads to a frequent utilization for monomodal CT registration (see Table 2.1). Moreover, the demons-based forces introduced by Thirion [1995] are closely related to SSD [Pennec et al. 1999] and often called Normalized SSD (NSSD).

Cross Correlation If a linear relationship exist between the intensity values of reference and template image, Normalized Cross Correlation (NCC) is to be preferred as similarity measure [Hill et al. 2001]. It is therefore often used for multimodal registration but also to overcome intensity changes caused by tissue compression in lung registration [Avants et al. 2008].

Mutual Information Mutual Information (MI) as a similarity measure is adapted from information theory and was proposed for image registration by Viola and Wells [1995]. It is aimed at minimizing the joint entropy of the greyvalues of both images (interpreted as random variables) and thereby maximizing the dependency between the images. To obtain overlap invariance, an extension to Normalized MI (NMI) was proposed by Studholme et al. [1999]. Even though primarily applied to multimodal registration, it can also be used for lung alignment [Modat et al. 2010a].

Normalized Gradient Field Mutual information is highly non-convex and often has numerous local minima [Modersitzki 2004]. To overcome this drawback, Haber and Modersitzki [2006] proposed to align images based on their gradients rather than intensities. The according distance measure is called Normalized Gradient Field (NGF) and applied to lung registration in [Rühaak et al. 2013].

Task-specific constraints In several approaches, specific properties of lung anatomy are modeled as an (additional) distance metric. Cao et al. [2010a] formulate the Sum of Squared Vesselness Measure Differences (SSVMD) to explicitly align the low-contrasted vasculature of the lung. Additionally, the Sum of Squared Tissue Volume Differences (SSTVD) is used to account for the intensity variations in lung CT images during respiration. With the same purpose, a mass-preserving registration is presented in [Yin et al. 2009] and [Gorbunova et al. 2012].

2.1.4 Algorithmic solutions

For minimizing the functional (2.1), different strategies are followed in the literature, which are briefly summarized in the following. For a mathematically profound overview, the reader is referred to [Clarenz et al. 2006].

Algorithm-driven approaches In several approaches – most prominently the demons registration proposed by [Thirion 1995] – the algorithm is driven by the aim of matching images rather then explicitly solving (2.1) or a similar functional.[2] Here, registration is usually performed using an iterative two-step approach: First the transformation is varied a bit in a certain direction, for example inspired by the computation of the optical flow [Horn and Schunck 1981]. Second, the optimized transformation is smoothed, most commonly using a Gaussian filtering. In [Han 2010] and [Heinrich et al. 2012], similar *pair-and-smooth* procedures consisting of an iterative feature or template matching and smoothing are applied.

Variational approaches Most commonly, the energy functional (2.1) is minimized using the calculus of variations. More precisely, the Euler-Lagrange equation (ELE) of the energy, which constitutes a necessary condition for a (local) minimum, is analytically derived. Then, an optimization method like the gradient descent (GD) is employed to iteratively find a transformation for which the condition is fulfilled. Finally, the derived scheme is discretized. This approach is therefore also called an *optimize-then-discretize* strategy.

Discrete optimization approaches The *discretize-then-optimize* strategy can be seen as the more intuitive one, as the images at hand are always discrete. Here, the energy functional is discretized in a first step to obtain a finite optimization problem. As a consequence, well-known numerical optimization techniques like the Gauss-Newton or Broyden–Fletcher–Goldfarb–Shanno (BFGS) methods can be applied to solve the registration problem [Nocedal and Wright 2006]. This approach is pursued for example in [Olesch et al. 2009; Rühaak et al. 2011]. Other discrete optimization techniques include Markov Random Fields (MRF), which are employed in [Heinrich et al. 2012].

2.2 Open-source implementations

The registration community is blessed with a huge number of open-source implementations, which can be utilized to solve various problems. In the following section, a brief overview is given.

---

[2] In case of demons registration, however, the ad-hoc algorithm can be reduced to minimizing (2.1), as derived in [Modersitzki 2004].

ITK   The Insight Segmentation and Registration Toolkit (ITK) is a powerful C++ frame-work for various tasks of image processing, such as registration, segmentation and image enhancement. It provides a flexible implementation of linear registration algorithms, however, the possibilities for non-linear registration are limited. This is in the focus of current developments [Avants et al. 2012]. Major parts of the algorithms developed in this thesis are implemented as modules for the ITK framework.

ANTS   The Advanced Normalization Tools (ANTS) are developed at the Penn Image Computing and Science Lab of the University of Pennsylvania, Philadelphia, US and can be accessed under http://www.picsl.upenn.edu/ANTS/. The framework provides flex-ible tools for elastic and B-spline registration with a variety of distance measures (NCC, MI, SSD, etc.). Moreover, transformations can be restricted to diffeomorphisms based on static and time-dependent velocity fields [Avants et al. 2008].

Nifty Reg   The Nifty Reg package is provided by the University College London, London, UK (see http://sourceforge.net/projects/niftyreg/). It implements affine and FFD-based algorithms using NMI as metric. The focus is on a performant implementation using hardware acceleration [Modat et al. 2010b].

elastix   The elastix framework (see http://elastix.isi.uu.nl/) provides multiple registration algorithms based on affine and B-spline transformations and various metrics (SSD, CC, MI, NMI, etc.) [Klein et al. 2010].

FAIR   The Flexible Algorithms for Image Registration (FAIR) toolbox is a package written in MATLAB primarily thought for academic purposes [Modersitzki 2009]. Discrete optimization techniques are followed in this implementation. It can be assessed via http://www.siam.org/books/fa06/.

2.3 Discussion

The presented overview illustrates the widely spread possibilities to approach the task of image registration. Even though evaluation studies have been conducted to assess accuracy of different methods, it is difficult to determine superior methods because only complete algorithms are compared. Therefore, it is not possible to deduce a meaningful ranking of the single components. For example, NSSD, NCC as well as NMI have all been used in top-ranked approaches. Moreover, minor differences in the implementation, pre-processing steps and the pre-registration have a major impact on the results.

To deal with this problem, a flexible framework for image registration is employed in this work. Its modular design allows a direct comparison of the components like transformation, distance measure and regularization. The algorithm found to be optimal then serves as basis for subsequent examinations.

Chapter 3

Variational image registration

In this chapter, a flexible registration framework is formulated based on the preceding overview on current methods for the registration of thoracic CT images. Here, the focus is on dense transformation models and calculus of variations to solve the problem. However, the framework enables the integration of various well-established formulations of the similarity measure and the smoothing term as introduced in Chapter 2. In contrast to evaluation studies such as [Murphy et al. 2011b], this modular design allows the comparison of different approaches on the level of their components, and not whole registration algorithms. This is performed in Chapter 7.2 with the goal of identifying the best-suited algorithm for lung registration. The presented framework also forms the basis for the examinations and extensions presented in the following chapters.

Largely following the notation introduced by Modersitzki [2004], a registration framework based on energy minimization is presented in Section 3.1 and a numerical solution of the problem is derived. After various approaches for defining the main components of the framework – distance measure and regularization scheme – have already been outlined in Chapter 2, the specific terms used in this framework are detailed in Section 3.2 and 3.3, respectively. The subsequent Section 3.4 aims at presenting an extension of the registration framework that is used to ensure the transformation to be diffeomorphic, that means differentiable and invertible. In the concluding Sections 3.5 and 3.6, the functionality of the different components of the framework is experimentally demonstrated and the main findings are discussed.

3.1 Image registration as a minimization problem

Given two d-dimensional images[1] called reference image $R : \Omega \to \mathbb{R}$ and template image $T : \Omega \to \mathbb{R}$ with the image domain[2] $\Omega \subset \mathbb{R}^d$, the registration problem is formulated as

---

[1] A more formal definition of digital images is given in Appendix A.
[2] In this work, $\Omega = \Omega_R = \Omega_T$ is assumed. This can always be ensured by applying a pre-registration.

the task of finding a "plausible" transformation $\varphi : \Omega \to \Omega$ that maps the domain of the template image to the domain of the reference image. The optimal transformation $\hat{\varphi}$ is determined by solving the minimization problem

$$\hat{\varphi} = \arg\min_{\varphi} \mathcal{J}^{Reg}[\varphi] \,, \tag{3.1}$$

with the energy functional

$$\mathcal{J}^{Reg}[\varphi] := \mathcal{D}[R, T; \varphi] + \alpha \mathcal{S}[\varphi] \,. \tag{3.2}$$

As in the previous chapter, $\mathcal{D}$ is a distance measure quantifying the (dis-)similarity between reference and transformed template image. The plausibility of the motion field is controlled by the regularizer $\mathcal{S}$, which is applied to smooth the transformation and thereby avoiding discontinuities like gaps or foldings. The parameter $\alpha \in \mathbb{R}^+$ weights the influence of the regularization. If not required for comprehension, the superscript of $\mathcal{J}^{Reg}$ is omitted in the following.

In the basic framework presented in this section, the transformation φ is assumed to be given by a displacement $\boldsymbol{u} : \Omega \to \mathbb{R}^d$ via $\varphi(\boldsymbol{x}) := \boldsymbol{x} - \boldsymbol{u}(\boldsymbol{x})$. Here, an Eulerian view is followed, that means a point in the reference image is mapped to the corresponding point in the template image. Since optimizing φ is equivalent to optimizing $\boldsymbol{u}$, $\mathcal{J}[\boldsymbol{u}]$ is used as a synonym for $\mathcal{J}[\varphi]$ in the following.

In this work, an optimize-then-discretize strategy as outlined in Chapter 2 is followed. First, in Section 3.1.1, the calculus of variations is utilized to formulate the Euler-Lagrange equation of the energy functional. This equation gives a necessary condition for the existence of a (local) minimum. In Section 3.1.2, the Euler-Lagrange equation is then discretized and a numeric approach is presented to iteratively determine a solution of the problem.

The section at hand is intended to only give an overview on the methodology; Much more thorough and mathematically detailed analyses can be found for example in [Modersitzki 2004; Heldmann 2006; Kabus 2006].

3.1.1 The Euler-Lagrange equation

Assuming the existence of a solution $\hat{\boldsymbol{u}}$ of the registration problem (3.1), the function $\Upsilon : \mathbb{R} \to \mathbb{R}$ with

$$\Upsilon(\epsilon) := \mathcal{J}[\hat{\boldsymbol{u}} + \epsilon \boldsymbol{v}]$$

is known to have a (local) minimum at $\Upsilon(0)$ for all test functions $\boldsymbol{v} : \mathbb{R}^d \to \mathbb{R}^d$. Consequently, the first order derivative has to vanish at $\epsilon = 0$:

$$0 = \Upsilon'(0) = \left. \frac{d\mathcal{J}[\hat{\boldsymbol{u}} + \epsilon \boldsymbol{v}]}{d\epsilon} \right|_{\epsilon=0} \,.$$

This term is called the Gâteaux derivative or first variation of $\mathcal{J}$ in the direction of $\boldsymbol{v}$, which is defined as

$$\delta\mathcal{J}[\boldsymbol{u};\boldsymbol{v}] := \left.\frac{d\mathcal{J}[\boldsymbol{u}+\epsilon\boldsymbol{v}]}{d\epsilon}\right|_{\epsilon=0} = \lim_{\epsilon\to 0}\frac{1}{\epsilon}\Big(\mathcal{J}[\boldsymbol{u}+\epsilon\boldsymbol{v}] - \mathcal{J}[\boldsymbol{u}]\Big). \tag{3.3}$$

If $\hat{\boldsymbol{u}}$ is a local minimizer of $\mathcal{J}$ (also called a stationary point of $\mathcal{J}$), then

$$\delta\mathcal{J}[\hat{\boldsymbol{u}};\boldsymbol{v}] = 0 \tag{3.4}$$

for all variations $\boldsymbol{v}$. This condition is the Euler-Lagrange equation of $\mathcal{J}$. Inserting the terms for distance measure and regularization further yields

$$\delta\mathcal{J}[\boldsymbol{u};\boldsymbol{v}] = \delta\mathcal{D}[\boldsymbol{u};\boldsymbol{v}] + \alpha\,\delta\mathcal{S}[\boldsymbol{u};\boldsymbol{v}]. \tag{3.5}$$

The next step aims at finding a displacement $\boldsymbol{u}$ (and a transformation φ, respectively) that fulfills the condition (3.4). Given the L^2 inner product

$$\langle\boldsymbol{u},\boldsymbol{v}\rangle_{L^2(\Omega)} := \int_\Omega \boldsymbol{u}(\boldsymbol{x})\cdot\boldsymbol{v}(\boldsymbol{x})\,d\boldsymbol{x},$$

$\nabla\mathcal{J}$ is called the *gradient* of $\mathcal{J}$ if

$$\delta\mathcal{J}[\boldsymbol{u};\boldsymbol{v}] = \langle\nabla\mathcal{J}[\boldsymbol{u}],\boldsymbol{v}\rangle_{L^2(\Omega)}.$$

Accordingly, $\nabla\mathcal{J}[\hat{\boldsymbol{u}}] = 0$ is a condition for a minimizer $\hat{\boldsymbol{u}}$ of $\mathcal{J}$.

Assembling the specific terms for $\mathcal{D}$ and $\mathcal{S}$ yields together with (3.5) the expression

$$\nabla\mathcal{J}[\boldsymbol{u}] = \boldsymbol{f}(\boldsymbol{u}) - \alpha\mathcal{A}[\boldsymbol{u}],$$

where the force term $\boldsymbol{f}$ corresponds to the distance measure and $\mathcal{A}$ is a linear differential operator related to the regularizer. The precise Gâteaux derivatives of the specific distance measure and regularizer used in this work are derived in the dedicated sections. It is known from optimization theory that the negative gradient points in the direction of the steepest descent. By introducing an artificial time t and additionally letting $\boldsymbol{u}$ depend on that time parameter, a gradient descent process is defined by

$$\partial_t\boldsymbol{u} = -\nabla\mathcal{J}[\boldsymbol{u}] = -\big(\boldsymbol{f}(\boldsymbol{u}) - \alpha\mathcal{A}[\boldsymbol{u}]\big). \tag{3.6}$$

At a stationary point $\hat{\boldsymbol{u}}$ of $\mathcal{J}$, the gradient vanishes and the evolution converges with $\partial_t\hat{\boldsymbol{u}} = 0$. As detailed by Heldmann [2006], a stady-state solution can be interpreted from a physical point of view as a system in equilibrum between forces $\boldsymbol{f}(\boldsymbol{u})$ acting on the system and the reaction $-\alpha\mathcal{A}[\boldsymbol{u}]$ of the system.

To iteratively solve equation (3.6), an (explicit) forward Euler step can be applied by discretizing the time with a step size $\tau \in \mathbb{R}^+$ and setting $t_{k+1} = t_k + \tau$, with k being the iteration index. A finite difference approximation of $\partial_t \boldsymbol{u}$ yields

$$\boldsymbol{u}^{(k+1)} = \boldsymbol{u}^{(k)} - \tau \left(\boldsymbol{f}(\boldsymbol{u}^{(k)}) - \alpha \mathcal{A}[\boldsymbol{u}^{(k)}] \right) \tag{3.7}$$

with $\boldsymbol{u}^{(k)} := \boldsymbol{u}(t_k)$ and any given initialization $\boldsymbol{u}^{(0)}$. While this allows a straightforward implementation, explicit schemes are known to be unstable and suffer from severe restrictions on the step size τ (see Sections 3.3.1.1 and 3.3.2.1 for details). However, an implicit backwards scheme cannot be used directly due to the non-linearity of $\boldsymbol{f}(\boldsymbol{u})$. As an alternative, $\boldsymbol{f}(\boldsymbol{u}^{(k+1)})$ can be approximated by the force $\boldsymbol{f}(\boldsymbol{u}^{(k)})$ of the previous step and the semi-implicit scheme

$$(Id - \tau \alpha \mathcal{A}) [\boldsymbol{u}^{(k+1)}] = \boldsymbol{u}^{(k)} - \tau \boldsymbol{f}(\boldsymbol{u}^{(k)}) \quad . \tag{3.8}$$

can be used, where Id is the identity mapping. The computational complexity of solving this partial differential equation essentially depends on the differential operator $\mathcal{A}$. The choice between explicit and semi-implicit scheme can therefore only be made with regard to the specific regularizer and will be discussed in the corresponding sections.

3.1.2 Discretization and stability considerations

To compute a solution of the registration problem, the partial differential equations (3.7) and (3.8) first have to be discretized. The domain Ω is discretized according to the image grid of $\vec{R}$ as described in Appendix A. Given a lexicographic ordering, this yields the N grid points $\boldsymbol{x}_1, \ldots, \boldsymbol{x}_N$, where $N = N_1 \cdots N_d$ is the total number of voxels. The l-th component of the displacement $\boldsymbol{u} = (u_1, \ldots, u_d)^T$ can then be assembled in the vector

$$\vec{U}_l := (u_l(\boldsymbol{x}_j))_{j=1,\ldots,N} \in \mathbb{R}^N , \quad l = 1, \ldots, d .$$

The complete field is collected in the $Nd \times 1$ vector $\vec{U} := (\vec{U}_1^T, \ldots, \vec{U}_d^T)^T$. Correspondingly, $\vec{F}$ is the discrete force field built of the values of $\boldsymbol{f}$ at grid points. The differential operator $\mathcal{A}$ is discretized using finite differences, yielding the $Nd \times Nd$ matrix[3] $A^{Nd,Nd}$. This procedure is detailed for specific regularizers in Section 3.3.

Putting all together, the discrete explicit solution scheme (3.7) reads

$$\begin{aligned}
\vec{U}^{(k+1)} &= (I + \tau \alpha A) \, \vec{U}^{(k)} - \tau \vec{F}^{(k)} \\
&= (I + \tau \alpha A)^{k+1} \, \vec{U}^{(0)} - \sum_{i=0}^{k} \tau \, (I + \tau \alpha A)^i \, \vec{F}^{(k-i)} ,
\end{aligned} \tag{3.9}$$

---

[3] To enhance readability, the index indicating the size of the matrix is omitted in the following, if not required for comprehension.

with I denoting the $Nd \times Nd$ identity matrix. As apparent from the second row of equation (3.9), the solution only converges to a constant steady-state and is therefore stable if all eigenvalues of the matrix $(I + \tau \alpha A)$ lie in the interval $[-1, 1]$. To this end, to maintain stability, a step size $\tau \leq \tau_{max}$ has to be chosen such that this condition is fulfilled, with τ_{max} depending on the maximal eigenvalue λ_{max} of the matrix A. This entails the aforementioned restrictions on the step size τ, which lead to slow convergence of the algorithm and an increased risk of getting stuck in a local minimum.

Discretizing the semi-implicit scheme (3.8) leads to the systems of linear equations

$$(I - \tau \alpha A)\, \vec{U}^{(k+1)} = \vec{U}^{(k)} - \tau \vec{F}^{(k)} \,. \tag{3.10}$$

While this scheme has no restrictions on τ, solving the linear system is not feasible for every matrix A. However, optimization techniques exist for specific regularizers and these will be discussed in Section 3.3.

The final registration algorithm for both the explicit and the semi-implicit scheme is summarized in Algorithm 3.1. Note that for the explicit scheme, the algorithm (last step: smoothing) slightly deviates from (3.7), where the smoothing is carried out before force computation. This has practical reasons and a negligible effect on the results.

Algorithm 3.1 Non-linear registration.

1: Set $k = 0$ and set $\vec{U}^{(0)}$ to zero.
2: **repeat**
3:    Compute the force $\vec{F}^{(k)}$.   ▷ Section 3.2
4:    Let $\vec{U}^{(k)} \leftarrow \vec{U}^{(k)} - \tau \vec{F}^{(k)}$.
5:    Let $\vec{U}^{(k)} \leftarrow (I + \tau \alpha A)\, \vec{U}^{(k)}$ (explicit) or
      solve $(I - \tau \alpha A)\, \vec{U}^{(k+1)} = \vec{U}^{(k)}$ (semi-implicit).   ▷ Section 3.3
6:    Let $k \leftarrow k + 1$.
7: **until** algorithm converges or $k = k_{max}$.

3.1.3 Multi-scale registration

Multi-scale approaches (also called multi-resolution or multi-level approaches[4]) are commonly applied to enhance computational efficiency of registration algorithms and reduce the risk of getting stuck in a local minimum. Based on scale-space theory developed by Witkin [1983] and Lindeberg [1990], they aim at getting a preliminary

---

[4] Multi-scale approaches should not be confused with multigrid methods [Briggs et al. 2000], which are not in the focus of this work.

coarse approximation of the transformation by registering "simplified" (that means blurred) versions of the images and then recursively adding more and more detail to achieve a finer matching. To this end, the original image $I(\boldsymbol{x})$ is embedded in a family of derived images – the scale-space of the image – spanned by a scaling parameter that describes the level of detail. The most reasonable choice is the *Gaussian scale-space*

$$I(\boldsymbol{x}, \sigma) := I(\boldsymbol{x}) * G_\sigma$$

with the scaling parameter σ denoting the standard deviation of the Gaussian kernel G_σ. This approach helps to avoid local minima during the minimization process.

Moreover, to reduce computational effort, an efficient way to construct $I(\boldsymbol{x}, \sigma)$ is a recursive downsampling of the image after convolution with a Gaussian kernel to avoid aliasing effects (for example, resampling to half resolution in each dimension for $\sigma = 1.0$ according to the Nyquist-Shannon sampling theorem). The registration is then first performed with the coarsest (that means smallest) images and the resulting transformation is up-sampled to serve as initialization for the registration on the next scale.

3.2 Distance Measures

In this section, different possibilities for defining the distance measures $\mathcal{D}$ are regarded, which quantifies the dissimilarity between reference and transformed template image. The appropriate choice for this metric depends on the specific application, in particular the modality of the images. Keeping the application of lung registration in mind and therefore focussing on monomodal registration, different possibilities for defining the similarity metric are detailed in the following.

3.2.1 (Normalized) Sum of Squared Differences

The most straightforward and intuitive approach for defining the dissimilarity between two images is based on the assumption that an object has the same intensity in both images, subject only to Gaussian noise. If this condition is met, the optimal metric is the *Sum of Squared Differences* (SSD)

$$\mathcal{D}^{SSD}[R, T; \varphi] := \frac{1}{2} \int_\Omega \left(R(\boldsymbol{x}) - T \circ \varphi(\boldsymbol{x}) \right)^2 d\boldsymbol{x} \,. \tag{3.11}$$

The validity of the assumption of constant greyvalues will be discussed in Section 7.2.1.1 for the specific application of lung registration in CT images.

Deriving the Euler-Lagrange equation for $\mathcal{D}$ as detailed in Section B.1.1 yields the force term

$$f^{SSD}(u) := (R - T \circ \varphi) \nabla(T \circ \varphi) \, .$$

In his work about *demon-based registration*, Thirion [1995] introduced alternative formulations of the force term. In contrast to the SSD-based force,

$$f^{act}(u) := \frac{R - T \circ \varphi}{\|\nabla(T \circ \varphi)\|^2 + \gamma \cdot (R - T \circ \varphi)^2} \nabla(T \circ \varphi) \tag{3.12}$$

induces stronger forces in regions with low image contrast by utilizing the normalized gradient. Therefore, this term is commonly called the *Normalized Sum of Squared Differences* (NSSD). An $\gamma \neq 0$ is used to prevent instability in regions with a contrast close to zero. In analogy to many publications, $\gamma := 1/\bar{h}^2$ with $\bar{h}^2$ denoting the mean squared spacing of the image is used in this work [Thirion 1998; Vercauteren et al. 2007].

While f^{act} causes an *active force* "pushing" the template image to fit the reference image, the term

$$f^{pas}(u) := \frac{R - T \circ \varphi}{\|\nabla R\|^2 + \gamma \cdot (R - T \circ \varphi)^2} \nabla R \tag{3.13}$$

acts as a *passive force* "pulling" the template image. This term provides a computational benefit because the gradients remain fixed and do not have to be calculated in each iteration. Active and passive forces are illustrated in Figure 3.1.

As a combination of both terms,

$$f^{dual}(u) := \frac{(R - T \circ \varphi) \cdot (\nabla R + \nabla(T \circ \varphi))}{\|\nabla R + \nabla(T \circ \varphi)\|^2 + \gamma \cdot (R - T \circ \varphi)^2} \tag{3.14}$$

was proposed. Both f^{act} and f^{pas} are closely related to the second order approximation of the SSD gradient [Pennec et al. 1999]. Still, no publication quoting the energy corresponding to these terms for the particular choice of γ is known to the author of this work.

3.2.2 Other distance measures

As detailed in Chapter 2, a variety of distance measures have been applied in lung registration besides the (Normalized) SSD. In general, these are compatible with the presented framework and can be employed without major adjustments. For example, (Normalized) Mutual Information (NMI) [Maes et al. 1997], Cross Correlation (CC) [Kim and Fessler 2004] or the Normalized Gradient Flow (NGF) [Haber and Modersitzki 2006] are applied in very similar settings. A comprehensive overview on distance measures in a variational framework is for example given in [Hermosillo et al. 2002]. Also, additional

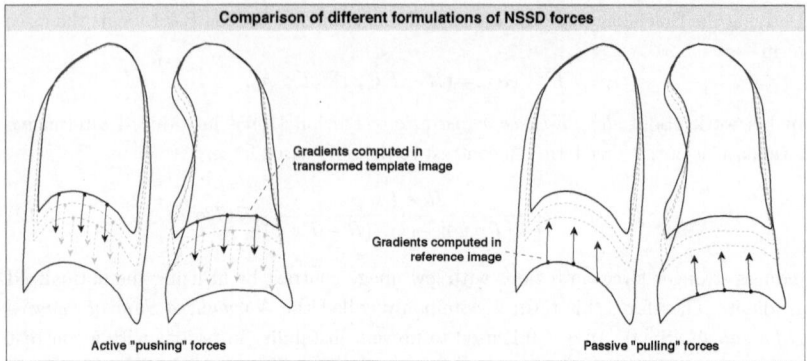

Figure 3.1: Comparison of active (left) and passive forces (right). Active forces $\boldsymbol{f}^{act}$ are based on the gradients of the transformed template image, which have to be recalculated in each iteration. In contrast to this, gradients of the reference image as used for the computation of $\boldsymbol{f}^{pas}$ remain fixed. Illustration taken from [Schmidt-Richberg et al. 2009a].

distance terms can be appended to enforce a conservation of mass [Gorbunova et al. 2012] or an improved vessel alignment [Cao et al. 2010a]. However, these measures are not further regarded in the context of this work.

3.3 Regularizer

In the following section, common regularization techniques are introduced, namely diffusion and elastic regularization. Moreover, a Gaussian smoothing is regarded, which is not directly compatible to the formulation of the registration problem (3.2) but is often applied in practice (see Chapter 2).

For all regularizers, stability properties of the explicit solution scheme are examined and methods for a semi-implicit solution are referred to.

3.3.1 Diffusion regularization

Diffusion is intuitively understood as the physical process that equilibrates concentration differences without creating or destroying mass. This principle can be mathematically expressed by the *diffusion equation*

$$\partial_t u = \nabla (D \nabla u) ,$$

where $u = u(\boldsymbol{x}, t)$ is a function describing a physical property – for example, the temperature of a material or the concentration of a gas – and D denotes the diffusion tensor that steers the diffusion process. This equation is used to model many physical transport processes as for example – in the context of heat transfer – the heat equation. Diffusion filtering is commonly used as a technique for smoothing images. Its application as a regularizer in image registration is realized, for example, by Fischer and Modersitzki [2002]. While it is lacking a physical motivation from the field of material deformation, it allows a very simple and efficient implementation. The isotropic diffusion equation can be derived from the energy functional

$$\mathcal{S}^{diff}[\boldsymbol{u}] := \frac{1}{2} \sum_{l=1}^{d} \int_{\Omega} \|\nabla u_l(\boldsymbol{x})\|^2 \, d\boldsymbol{x}, \tag{3.15}$$

which aims at penalizing large gradients of the displacement. Derivation of the Euler-Lagrange equation as detailed in Appendix B.1.1 yields

$$\mathcal{A}^{diff}[\boldsymbol{u}] = \Delta \boldsymbol{u}$$

for the optimization, with $\Delta \boldsymbol{u} := (\Delta u_1, \ldots, \Delta u_d)^T$ and $\Delta u_l := \nabla \cdot \nabla u_l$ denoting the Laplace operator of a function u_l. This corresponds to the diffusion equation with D being the identity. The steady-state solution for diffusion registration yields the Poisson equation $\Delta \boldsymbol{u} = \boldsymbol{f}$, which – from a physical point of view – can be interpreted as the stationary heat equation for a system with heat source $\boldsymbol{f}$.

3.3.1.1 Stability properties of the explicit scheme

To formulate discretization of the Laplace operator, the 1D case is examined first. Approximating Δ using finite differences yields the $N \times N$ matrix $A^{N,N} = (a_{ij})$ with

$$a_{ij} = \begin{cases} \frac{1}{h^2} & j \in \{i-1, i+1\}, \\ -\frac{2}{h^2} & j = i, \\ 0 & \text{else} \end{cases} \tag{3.16}$$

with h denoting the pixel spacing. Neumann boundary conditions are incorporated by setting $a_{11} = a_{NN} = -\frac{1}{h^2}$. Following the Gerschgorin circle theorem, all eigenvalues λ_i of a square matrix $M = (m_{ij})$ lie in *discs* with the radius $r_i := \sum_{j \neq i} |m_{ij}|$ and the center $c_i := m_{ii}$ [Gerschgorin 1931]. For the specific matrix A, this leads to $\lambda_{max} \in [c_i - r_i, c_i + r_i] = [-\frac{4}{h^2}, 0]$. Accordingly, a step size $\tau_{max} = \frac{h^2}{2\alpha}$ has to be chosen to maintain numerical stability.

In the d-dimensional case, each component of the displacement field can be regularized independently because here, $A^{diff} = \text{diag}(A_1^{diff}, \ldots, A_d^{diff})$ is block diagonal. It is

$$\vec{U}_l^{(k+1)} = \left(I + \tau\alpha \sum_{m=1}^{d} A_m \right) \vec{U}_l^{(k)} - \tau \vec{F}_l^{(k)} \tag{3.17}$$

for all $l = 1, \ldots, d$. Here, the matrix A_l^{diff} is constructed with matrices A_m that correspond to the derivatives along the m-th coordinate axis. These matrices can be assembled using the Kronecker product. In the tree-dimensional case this yields for example

$$A_1 = I^{N_3,N_3} \otimes I^{N_2,N_2} \otimes A^{N_1,N_1}$$
$$A_2 = I^{N_3,N_3} \otimes A^{N_2,N_2} \otimes I^{N_1,N_1}$$
$$A_3 = A^{N_3,N_3} \otimes I^{N_2,N_2} \otimes I^{N_1,N_1} .$$

using the lexicographic order introduced in Appendix A. Again applying Gershgorin's circle theorem reveals the maximal time step

$$\tau_{max} = \frac{1}{\alpha} \left(\sum_{m=1}^{d} \frac{2}{h_m^2} \right)^{-1} ,$$

with h_m denoting the spacing in direction of the m-th coordinate axis, which simplifies to $\tau_{max} = \frac{h^2}{2d\alpha}$ for isotropic spacing.

3.3.1.2 Diffusion regularization with Fast Explicit Diffusion

To circumvent the aforementioned disadvantages of the explicit solution schemes, Grewenig et al. [2010] recently proposed *Fast Explicit Diffusion* (FED) for solving diffusion problems. The approach is based on the observation, that a box filtering

$$(B_{2n+1}(\vec{U}))_j := \frac{1}{2n+1} \sum_{k=-n}^{n} U_{j+k}$$

of size $2n + 1$, $n \in \mathbb{N}$ at index j can be approximated by a cycle of n explicit linear diffusion steps

$$B_{2n+1} = \prod_{i=0}^{n-1} (I + \tau_i A)$$

where A is a finite difference approximation of Δ as defined in (3.16) and the varying time steps are given by

$$\tau_i = \frac{\tau_{max}}{2 \cos^2 \left(\pi \frac{2i+1}{4n+2} \right)} . \tag{3.18}$$

This is directly related to performing n iterations of diffusion regularization as defined in (3.9). Interestingly, since box filtering is stable, complete FED cycles are also stable even though individual steps massively violate the stability conditions. As a consequence, the stopping time

$$T(n) = \sum_{i=0}^{n-1} \tau_i$$

.

of one cycle is reached with considerably fewer iterations than when using fixed stable step sizes τ_{max}. Besides resulting in a faster convergence, this approach also has the advantage that local minima are avoided by occasional large steps. An FED cycle can either be specified by the number n of iterations per cycle or by the stopping time T. In that case, n is chosen to be the smallest number with $T(n) \geq T$. While the order of the time steps is arbitrary in theory, Grewenig et al. [2010] propose a reordering following Gentzsch [1980] to avoid instabilities introduced by numerical rounding.

Instead of approximating a box filter by simple diffusion steps, the approach can be adapted for arbitrary diffusion problems taking the maximal step size τ_{max} into account [Grewenig et al. 2010; Gwosdek et al. 2010].

3.3.1.3 Additive Operator Splitting for semi-implicit solution

Alternatively to using explicit schemes with restrictions on the time step, diffusion regularization can be efficiently solved using the semi-implicit scheme

$$\vec{U}_l^{(k+1)} = \left(I - \tau\alpha \sum_{m=1}^{d} A_m \right)^{-1} \vec{U}_l^{(k)} - \tau\vec{F}_l^{(k)} \qquad (3.19)$$

for $l = 1, \ldots, d$. A popular approach to solve this system is using *Additive Operator Splitting* (AOS) as proposed by Weickert et al. [1998]. The basic idea is to approximate (3.19) by

$$\vec{U}_l^{(k+1)} = \sum_{m=1}^{d} \left(I - \tau\alpha A_m \right)^{-1} \vec{U}_l^{(k)} - \tau\vec{F}_l^{(k)} . \qquad (3.20)$$

As proven for example in [Modersitzki 2004], the error made by this approximation is relative to τ^2 and therefore small for $\tau < 1$. The specific structure of the matrix A is now exploited to reach a high degree of factorization, leading to a very efficient implementation. First, equation (3.20) can be split in d subsystems

$$\left(I - \tau\alpha A_m \right) \vec{V}_{m,l}^{(k+1)} = \vec{U}_l^{(k)} - \tau\vec{F}_l^{(k)} , \quad m = 1, \ldots, d$$

with $\vec{U}_l = \frac{1}{d} \sum_{m=1}^{d} \vec{V}_{m,l}$. Using the properties of the Kronecker product, each of these equations can further be factorized in multiple systems of equations of size N_m, in each of which the matrix on the lefthand side has a tridiagonal structure. These systems can therefore easily be solved using the Thomas algorithm leading to a complexity of $\mathcal{O}(N)$. Diffusion regularization with AOS is summarized in Algorithm 3.2.

Algorithm 3.2 Diffusion regularization in 3D using Additive Operator Splitting (AOS). Here, $\vec{U}_l^{(j_1,j_2,j_3)\to x_m}$ denotes the vector in which the values of one row of the matrix U_l are collected in direction x_m starting at index (j_1, j_2, j_3) [Fischer and Modersitzki 2002].

1: Compute $B^{N_m} := \left(I - \tau\alpha A^{N_m,N_m}\right)$ and the LU decomposition for $m = 1$ to 3.
2: **for** $l = 1$ to 3 **do**
3:     Let $\vec{U}_l \leftarrow \vec{U}_l - \tau\vec{F}_l$.
4:     **for** $j_2 = 1$ to N_2 and $j_3 = 1$ to N_3 **do**
5:       Solve $B^{N_1} \cdot \vec{V}_{1,l}^{(1,j_2,j_3)\to x_1} = \vec{U}_l^{(1,j_2,j_3)\to x_1}$. $\triangleright$ Thomas algorithm
6:     **end for**
7:     **for** $j_1 = 1$ to N_1 and $j_3 = 1$ to N_3 **do**
8:       Solve $B^{N_2} \cdot \vec{V}_{2,l}^{(j_1,1,j_3)\to x_2} = \vec{U}_l^{(j_1,1,j_3)\to x_2}$. $\triangleright$ Thomas algorithm
9:     **end for**
10:    **for** $j_1 = 1$ to N_1 and $j_2 = 1$ to N_2 **do**
11:      Solve $B^{N_3} \cdot \vec{V}_{3,l}^{(j_1,j_2,1)\to x_3} = \vec{U}_l^{(j_1,j_2,1)\to x_3}$. $\triangleright$ Thomas algorithm
12:    **end for**
13:    Let $\vec{U}_l \leftarrow \frac{1}{3}\left(\vec{V}_{1,l} + \vec{V}_{2,l} + \vec{V}_{3,l}\right)$.
14: **end for**

3.3.2 Elastic regularization

Broit [1981] first proposed to regularize the deformation by minimizing its *linearized elastic potential*

$$\mathcal{S}^{elas}[\boldsymbol{u}] := \int_\Omega \frac{\mu}{4} \sum_{k,l=1}^{d} \left(\frac{\partial u_k}{\partial x_l} + \frac{\partial u_l}{\partial x_k}\right)^2 + \frac{\lambda}{2}(\operatorname{div}\boldsymbol{u})^2 \, d\boldsymbol{x}. \tag{3.21}$$

Here, μ and λ denote the so-called Lamé parameters, which describe the physical properties of the material. The physical motivation of elastic regularization is detailed for example in [Broit 1981; Modersitzki 2004].

As shown in [Kabus 2006], deriving the Euler-Lagrange equation leads to the Navier-Cauchy equation

$$\mathcal{A}^{elas}[\boldsymbol{u}] = \mu\Delta\boldsymbol{u} + (\mu + \lambda)\nabla\operatorname{div}\boldsymbol{u}.$$

If $\mu = 1$ and $\lambda = -1$, elastic smoothing reduces to diffusion regularization. However, this case is physically meaningless because it implies the Poisson's ratio $\nu = -\infty$.

3.3.2.1 Stability properties of the explicit scheme

In contrast to diffusion registration, regularization cannot be performed separately for each component in the elastic case because – as apparent from (3.21) – the motion in direction l has influence on the motion in direction k, with $l, k = 1, \ldots, d$ being dimension indices. A factorization as carried out in (3.17) for diffusion regularization is therefore not possible and the full system

$$\vec{U}^{(k+1)} = \left(I + \tau \alpha A^{elas} \right) \vec{U}^{(k)} - \tau \vec{F}^{(k)}$$

has to be solved, where the matrix A^{elas} is not block diagonal. The derivation of the precise matrix A^{elas} and the corresponding restrictions on the time step is found for example in [Kabus 2006; Modersitzki 2004]. Note that in addition to α, the stability of the explicit scheme also depends on the Lamé parameters μ and λ.

3.3.2.2 Semi-implicit solution in the frequency domain

Solving the equation

$$\vec{U}^{(k+1)} = \left(I - \tau \alpha A^{elas} \right)^{-1} \vec{U}^{(k)} - \tau \vec{F}^{(k)}$$

resulting from the semi-implicit scheme is not trivial because the matrix A^{elas} has a rich structure and can therefore not easily be inverted. Fischer and Modersitzki [1999], however, proposed a method to diagonalize A^{elas} using the *Fast Fourier Transformation* (FFT). The basic idea is to make $B := (I - \tau \alpha A^{elas})$ block-circulant by introducing periodic boundary conditions. Under this condition, a diagonal matrix D exists[5] with

$$D := F^H B F \,.$$

Here, $F = I^{d,d} \otimes F^{N_d} \otimes \cdots \otimes F^{N_1}$ is composed from the Fourier matrices $F^{N_l} \in \mathbb{C}^{N_l \times N_l}$ and F^H denotes the Hermitian conjugate of F. If $\det(B) \neq 0$, this can be reformulated to

$$B^{-1} = \left(F D F^H \right)^{-1} = F D^{-1} F^H \,.$$

Instead of inverting B, an efficient way for regularization is therefore transforming the updated displacement $\vec{U}_l - \tau \vec{F}_l$ into the frequency domain using FFT, solving the system in Fourier space with the easily invertible matrix D and transforming the result back into position space. Since the Fourier domain is location-independent, the system can be split in N subsystems of size $d \times d$. The final algorithm therefore has a complexity of $\mathcal{O}(N \log N)$ and is summarized in Algorithm 3.3. For details and a precise definition of the matrix D, the reader may refer to [Fischer and Modersitzki 1999; Modersitzki 2004].

---

[5] In fact, regarding the whole system, D is not diagonal but a block matrix composed of $d \times d$ diagonal matrices. However, it can still be inverted efficiently [Fischer and Modersitzki 1999].

Algorithm 3.3 Elastic regularization in 3D using matrix inversion in Fourier space. Here, $U_l^{(j_1, j_2, j_3)}$ denotes the value of U_l at index (j_1, j_2, j_3). The components $D_{k,l}$ of the matrix D are defined in [Fischer and Modersitzki 1999].

1: **for** $l = 1$ to 3 **do**
2:    Let $\vec{U}_l \leftarrow \vec{U}_l - \tau \vec{F}_l$.
3:    Compute $\tilde{U}_l = \texttt{fft3}(\vec{U}_l)$.
4: **end for**
5: **for** $j_1 = 1$ to N_1 and $j_2 = 1$ to N_2 and $j_3 = 1$ to N_3 **do**
6:    Solve

$$
\begin{pmatrix} \tilde{V}_1^{(j_1, j_2, j_3)} \\ \tilde{V}_2^{(j_1, j_2, j_3)} \\ \tilde{V}_3^{(j_1, j_2, j_3)} \end{pmatrix} = \begin{pmatrix} D_{1,1}^{(j_1, j_2, j_3)} & D_{1,2}^{(j_1, j_2, j_3)} & D_{1,3}^{(j_1, j_2, j_3)} \\ D_{2,1}^{(j_1, j_2, j_3)} & D_{2,2}^{(j_1, j_2, j_3)} & D_{2,3}^{(j_1, j_2, j_3)} \\ D_{3,1}^{(j_1, j_2, j_3)} & D_{3,2}^{(j_1, j_2, j_3)} & D_{3,3}^{(j_1, j_2, j_3)} \end{pmatrix}^{-1} \begin{pmatrix} \tilde{U}_1^{(j_1, j_2, j_3)} \\ \tilde{U}_2^{(j_1, j_2, j_3)} \\ \tilde{U}_3^{(j_1, j_2, j_3)} \end{pmatrix}.
$$

7: **end for**
8: **for** $l = 1$ to 3 **do**
9:    Compute $\vec{U}_l = \texttt{invfft3}(\tilde{V}_l)$.
10: **end for**

3.3.3 Gaussian smoothing

From a mathematical point of view, the Gaussian-based regularization is not directly compatible with the registration framework presented in this chapter – in particular with scheme (3.10) – as it does not stem from the minimization of an energy functional. However, as detailed for example in [Modersitzki 2004], Gaussian regularization is closely related to an analytical solution of the diffusion regularization (3.8). It is regarded in this context because of its wide employment in image registration since it is part of the classic demon-based registration [Thirion 1995, 1998].

Using Gaussian regularization, the scheme (3.10) is altered to

$$
U_l^{(k+1)} = \left(U_l^{(k)} - \tau F_l^{(k)} \right) * G_\sigma,
$$

where G_σ is a Gaussian kernel with standard deviation σ and F and U are the force and displacement field in discrete grid representation (see appendix A for details). The convolution can be performed with linear complexity $\mathcal{O}(N)$.

3.3.4 Other regularization approaches

Equivalently to the distance measures, other regularizers have been proposed that are compatible with the presented framework, most prominently the fluid regularization [Christensen 1994] or curvature-based approaches [Fischer and Modersitzki 2004]. In the context of this work, however, no additional regularization approaches are regarded.

3.4 Diffeomorphic registration

While transformations computed with the registration framework presented in Section 3.1 are generally smooth to a certain amount due to the regularization, additional demands are made on φ in some applications. In particular, invertibility of the displacement field is often required but not guaranteed by the classical registration scheme. It can be achieved by restricting the transformation to the group of diffeomorphisms.

A diffeomorphism $\varphi : \Omega \to \Omega$ is a differentiable bijective mapping, whose inverse φ^{-1} is differentiable as well. With Diff(Ω) the set of all diffeomorphisms over Ω is denoted. Note that Diff(Ω) is the underlying set of the group (Diff(Ω), $\circ$) with the composition $\circ$ as operation and the identity Id as neutral element. However, it is not closed under addition as used in (3.7) or (3.8) [Christensen et al. 1996]. Thus, these schemes cannot guarantee diffeomorphic transformations.

A diffeomorphic transformation can be modeled as the endpoint of the flow Φ over unit time $t \in [0,1]$, which is parameterized by a sufficiently smooth time-dependent velocity field $\boldsymbol{v} : \Omega \times [0,1] \to \mathbb{R}^d$ and the transport equation

$$\frac{\partial}{\partial t}\Phi(\boldsymbol{x},t) = \boldsymbol{v}(\Phi(\boldsymbol{x},t),t) \qquad \text{with} \qquad \Phi(\boldsymbol{x},0) = \boldsymbol{x}\,. \tag{3.22}$$

The specific conditions to the smoothness of $\boldsymbol{v}$ are discussed for example in [Dupuis et al. 1998; Trouvé 1998; Beg et al. 2005]. If they are satisfied, the transformation can be computed by

$$\varphi(\boldsymbol{x}) = \Phi(\boldsymbol{x},1) = \Phi(\boldsymbol{x},0) + \int_0^1 \boldsymbol{v}(\Phi(\boldsymbol{x},t),t)\,dt\,.$$

From a physical point of view, the integration can be interpreted as a description of the path a particle placed at point $\boldsymbol{x}$ covers subject to the time- and position-dependent velocity field $\boldsymbol{v}$.

The parametrization by velocity fields $\boldsymbol{v}(\boldsymbol{x},t)$ results in very time- and memory-consuming algorithms as presented for example in [Beg et al. 2005; Avants et al. 2006, 2008]. In recent works, however, the restriction to *stationary velocity fields* $\boldsymbol{v}(\boldsymbol{x})$ is examined, which define a one-parameter subgroup of the group of diffeomorphisms [Arsigny et al. 2006a; Arsigny 2006; Ehrhardt et al. 2011]. While diffeomorphisms parameterized by stationary fields have less degrees of freedom than the general case, they allow a much more efficient implementation and have been shown to be sufficiently versatile to describe the anatomical variations arising in medical applications [Ashburner 2007; Vercauteren et al. 2009; Hernandez et al. 2009].

To define an efficient registration algorithm it can further be exploited that the set of diffeomorphisms Diff(Ω) can be seen as a differentiable manifold, that means a topological space that is locally homeomorphic to Euclidean space. In addition to

---

Algorithm 3.4 Scaling and squaring algorithm for the computation of the vector field exponential [Arsigny et al. 2006a].

1: Choose n such that $2^{-n}v$ is close enough to zero, e.g. $\max \|2^{-n}v\| < \frac{\min_l h_l}{2}$
2: Let $\varphi(x) \leftarrow x + 2^{-n}v(x)$.   ▷ Scaling
3: **for** $i = 1$ to n **do**
4:     Let $\varphi(x) \leftarrow \varphi \circ \varphi(x)$.   ▷ Squaring
5: **end for**

---

the general group structure, $(\text{Diff}(\Omega), \circ)$ therefore is a lie group with an associated lie algebra $\mathfrak{g}$. The elements of the tangential space $\mathcal{T}_{Id}\text{Diff}(\Omega)$ at the neutral element build the underlying vector space of $\mathfrak{g}$. Interestingly, for diffeomorphisms parameterized by stationary vector fields, it is $v \in \mathcal{T}_{Id}\text{Diff}(\Omega)$ [Arsigny 2006]. Since lie algebra and lie group are connected by the *group exponential map*, this can be used to map an element v of the lie algebra to the corresponding element Φ of the lie group using

$$\exp : \mathcal{T}_{Id}\text{Diff}(\Omega) \to \text{Diff}(\Omega), \ \exp(tv) = \Phi(x, t) \,.$$

The transformation is then given by $\varphi(x) = \Phi(x, 1) = \exp(v(x))$. Furthermore, the inverse is defined by the exponential of the negative velocity field $\varphi^{-1}(x) = \exp(-v(x))$. Several algorithms for the computation of the exponential map – that means, the integration of the velocity field over time – are evaluated and compared to each other with respect to precision and efficiency in [Bossa et al. 2008]. Exploiting that $\exp(v) = \exp(n^{-1}v))^n$ for any integer $n \in \mathbb{N}$, Arsigny et al. [2006a] presented a particularly efficient approach for this purpose that requires only a small number of compositions. This scaling and squaring algorithm is summarized in Algorithm 3.4.

To restrict the registration framework to diffeomorphic mappings, a scalar product is defined in the tangential space by

$$\langle v, w \rangle_{\mathcal{T}_{Id}\text{Diff}(\Omega)} = \langle \mathcal{L}v, \mathcal{L}w \rangle_{L^2(\Omega)}$$

with a self-adjoint positive differential operator $\mathcal{L}$. With this, regularization of the velocity field can be interpreted as the search for paths with minimal the kinetic energy

$$\mathcal{S}[v] = \frac{1}{2} \int_0^1 \|v(\Phi(x, t))\|_{\mathcal{T}_{Id}\text{Diff}(\Omega)}^2 \, dt \,.$$

This is equivalent to the known regularization in L^2 space

$$\mathcal{S}[v] = \frac{1}{2} \int_0^1 \|\mathcal{L}v(\Phi(x, t))\|_{L^2(\Omega)}^2 \, dt \,,$$

given an appropriate choice of the operator $\mathcal{L}$ [Beg et al. 2005]. The resulting algorithm is given in Algorithm 3.5.

At this point, it should be noted that some theoretical problems remain unsolved. In particular, the precise requirements on the smoothness of the velocity field defined by the operator $\mathcal{L}$ remain unclear. Also, the Lie group $(\mathrm{Diff}(\Omega), \circ)$ is of infinite dimension and it is not clear, if general Lie group properties apply in this case. Moreover, the group exponential mapping is not surjective, that means there are elements of the group of diffeomorphisms that cannot be generated by (3.22). For more thorough discussions, the reader may refer to [Beg et al. 2005; Pennec 2006; Hernandez et al. 2009].

3.4.1 Symmetrization of forces

The direct availability of the inverse transformation when using a diffeomorphic registration approach can be exploited to symmetrize the force computation. By defining

$$\mathcal{D}^{sym}[R, T; \varphi] := \frac{1}{2} \left(\mathcal{D}[R, T; \varphi] + \mathcal{D}[T, R; \varphi^{-1}] \right) \tag{3.23}$$

it is requested that not only the transformed template image is similar to the reference image, but also the template image to the reference image deformed with the inverse transformation. When this term is applied, the result is independent of the choice of reference image.

Algorithm 3.5 Diffeomorphic non-linear registration.

1: Set $k = 0$ and set $\vec{V}^{(0)}$ and $\vec{U}^{(0)}$ to zero.
2: **repeat**
3:     Compute the force $\vec{F}^{(k)}$.   ▷ Section 3.2
4:     Let $\vec{V}^{(k)} \leftarrow \vec{V}^{(k)} - \tau \vec{F}^{(k)}$.
5:     Let $\vec{V}^{(k)} \leftarrow (I + \tau \alpha A) \vec{V}^{(k)}$ (explicit) or
        solve $(I - \tau \alpha A) \vec{V}^{(k)} = \vec{V}^{(k)}$ (semi-implicit).   ▷ Section 3.3
6:     Compute $\vec{U}^{(k)}$ from $\vec{V}^{(k)}$.   ▷ Algorithm 3.4
7:     Let $k \leftarrow k + 1$.
8: **until** algorithm converges or $k = k_{max}$.

3.5 Experiments

In the section at hand, different components of the registration framework are compared to each other. To demonstrate the basic functionality of these modules, registration is tested on synthetic images. The experiments are to be understood as a proof-of-concept study; An extensive quantitative evaluation using clinical data will follow in Chapter 7.

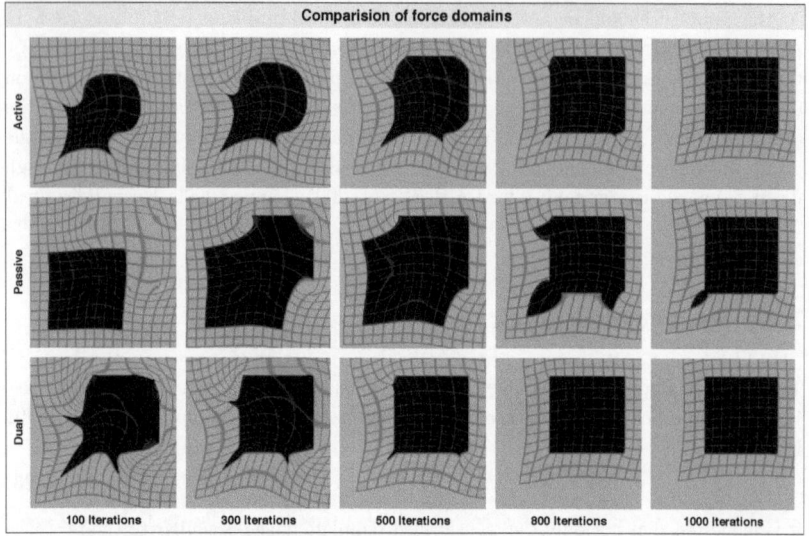

Figure 3.2: Comparison of active (top row), passive (center row), and dual forces (bottom row) in the course of 1000 iterations. Template and reference image are shown in Figure 3.4. All registrations are performed using semi-implicit diffusion regularization with $\tau = 1.0$ and $\alpha = 0.5$.

3.5.1 Comparison of force domains

In Section 3.11, different formulations of the NSSD-based forces have been presented following [Thirion 1998]. The principle difference is the image in which the forces are computed, which is referred to as force domain: While active forces $\boldsymbol{f}^{act}$ are computed using gradients of the transformed template image, passive forces $\boldsymbol{f}^{pas}$ are based on the gradients of the reference image (cf. Figure 3.1). Dual forces $\boldsymbol{f}^{dual}$ are a combination of active and passive forces.

In Figure 3.2, registration using these three types of forces is illustrated in the course of 1000 iterations. It is observed that the structure in the template image immediately moves in direction of the reference structure with active forces applied. Using passive forces, gradients are computed in the reference image and therefore start to evolve in the upper-right corner without instant effect on the template structure. Moreover, gradients in the reference image are fixed, that means passive forces are always pointing in the same direction that can only be altered by the regularization. This can lead to undesired effects as observed in particular at the lower-left corner of the structure. Dual forces combine the effects of active and passive forces.

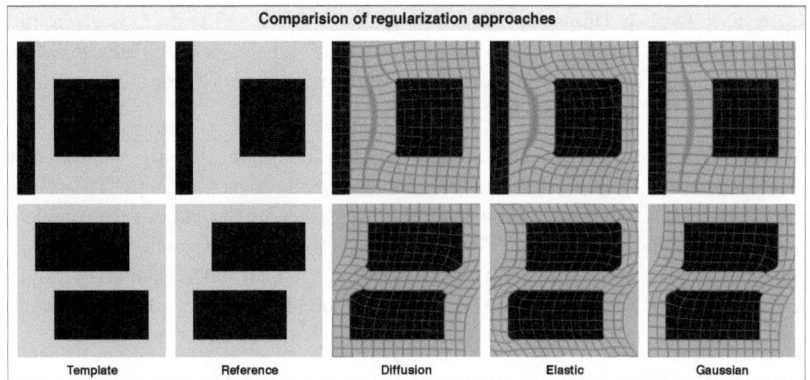

Figure 3.3: Comparison of diffusion ($\alpha = 0.5$), elastic ($\alpha = \mu = \lambda = 0.5$) and Gaussian regularization ($\sigma = 1.0$). Semi-implicit solution schemes are used for diffusion and elastic regularization. All experiments are performed with active forces, $\tau = 1.0$ and $k_{max} = 800$ iterations.

3.5.2 Comparison of regularizers

In Figure 3.3, the three approaches to regularization presented in Section 3.3 are compared to each other. The most obvious difference between diffusion and elastic regularization is caused by the periodic boundary conditions used for solving the Navier-Cauchy equation in Fourier space. This is particularly observed at the upper and lower boundaries in the second example. However, the effect of the underlying physical model of elastic regularization is also visible: In regions with high compression (that means "in front of" the moving objects), a sidewards-directed expansion is observed that aims at compensating for the aggregation of material in this region. Equivalently, the expansion arising "behind" objects causes deformations perpendicular to the direction of motion. This can be compared to the physical behavior expected when a rubber band is deformed. As anticipated, Gaussian regularization approximates diffusion regularization, differences are therefore negligible.

3.5.3 Comparison of solution schemes

In further experiments, the convergence behavior of explicit, semi-implicit and FED solution schemes are analyzed. For this, the *Mean Squared Difference* (MSD) of reference and deformed template image is plotted over the course of 1000 iterations in Figure 3.4. All registrations are performed using diffusion regularization with the same amount of smoothing ($\alpha = 0.5$) but the time step is adapted in each approach. For the explicit scheme, the theoretical limit for diffusion regularization with isotropic unit spacing of $\tau_{max} = 1/(\alpha 2d)$ is chosen. In the semi-implicit case, a time step of $\tau = 1.0$ is applicable.

Using Fast Explicit Diffusion, the stopping time T of one FED cycle is given and the number n of iterations per cycle as well as the time steps τ_i for each iteration are computed according to equation (3.18). In the experiments, three stopping times $T \in \{3.0, 5.0, 10.0\}$ are regarded.

As expected, the explicit scheme converges considerably slower than the semi-implicit and FED schemes. This is predominantly explained by the larger time steps. The graphs for FED clearly show that a stable state is only reached at the end of each complete cycle, which is the case every $n = 7$ iterations with $T = 3.0$ (this results in an average time step of $\bar{\tau}_i = 0.43$), every $n = 9$ iterations with $T = 5.0$ ($\bar{\tau}_i = 0.55$) and every $n = 13$ iterations with $T = 10.0$ ($\bar{\tau}_i = 0.77$). However, individual steps can be much larger, $T = 10.0$ for example implies time steps between 0.08 and 6.12.

In summary, FED exhibits a convergence behavior comparable to the semi-implicit scheme but with much lower computational cost per iteration.

3.5.4 Comparison of standard and diffeomorphic registration

To examine the effects of diffeomorphic registration with symmetric force term (3.23), the inverse consistency error is considered. In the ideal case, the composition $\varphi^{-1} \circ \varphi$ equals the identity. To compute the inverse transformation with the standard approach, reference and template image are exchanged in a second registration run. For the diffeomorphic registration, transformation and inverse are both obtained from the velocity field by $\varphi = \exp(\boldsymbol{v})$ and $\varphi^{-1} = \exp(-\boldsymbol{v})$, respectively (see Section 3.4).

The synthetic example illustrated in Figure 3.5 is challenging due to the high amount of compression/extension in the center region. This leads to discontinuities in the field using the standard approach, in particular a tearing effect in φ^{-1}. As a result, considerable divergences from identity arise in $\varphi^{-1} \circ \varphi$. For the diffeomorphic registration, however, the only differences are caused by interpolation and numerical approximation of the exponential map.

3.6 Discussion

In this chapter, a flexible framework for image registration was introduced. Using this approach, a problem-oriented adaption of the algorithm becomes possible by choosing specific modules of the algorithm, in particular the distance measure, the regularizer and the domain of the transformation. The experiments carried out in Section 3.5 demonstrate that the functionality of the modules is expedient. With this in mind, the framework will form the basis for application-specific extensions presented in the following chapters.

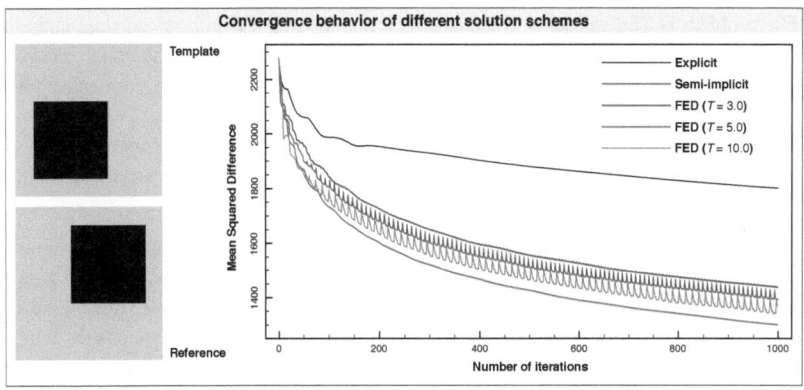

Figure 3.4: Comparison of the convergence of diffusion registration with explicit, semi-implicit and FED solution scheme. All registrations are performed with $\alpha = 0.5$. For the semi-implicit scheme, a time step of $\tau = 1.0$ is used, while the explicit scheme is performed with $\tau = \frac{1}{d}$, which maintains numerical stability. For FED, three examples with different times per FED cycle are given with $T = 3.0$ ($n = 7$ iterations per cycle), $T = 5.0$ ($n = 9$) and $T = 10.0$ ($n = 13$).

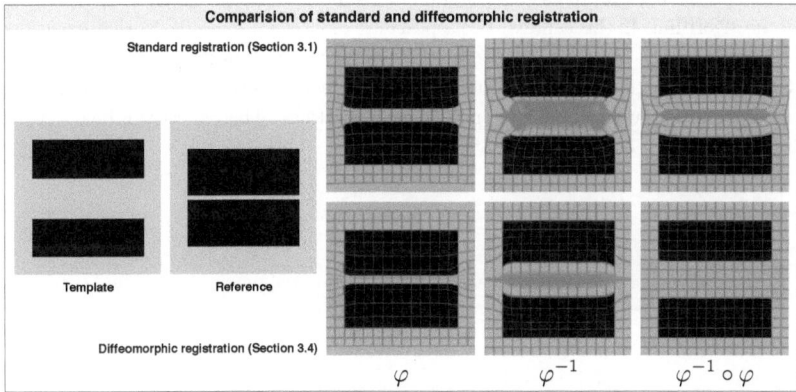

Figure 3.5: Comparison of standard (top row) and diffeomorphic registration (bottom row). All registrations are performed using semi-implicit diffusion regularization with $\tau = 1.0$, $\alpha = 0.5$ and $k_{max} = 800$. For the standard approach, the inverse transformation φ^{-1} is computed by exchanging reference and template image in a second registration run. Transformation and inverse are computed simultaneously in the diffeomorphic case (see Section 3.4).

The appropriate choice of the model parameters is of decisive importance for the algorithm. Primarily, the weight α (and equally μ, λ or σ for elastic and Gaussian regularization) influences the amount of smoothing and therefore has a major impact on the outcome. While the choice of the step width τ is intrinsic for the explicit scheme, the parameter has to be determined empirically in the semi-implicit case. The same holds for T if FED is utilized.

The problem is aggregated by the fact that a dependency exists between the maximal displacement in the force field $\max_\Omega \|f\|$ and τ. Using NSSD forces, the update vectors are guaranteed to be smaller than $\frac{h}{2}$ due to the normalization of the gradients. This does not hold for SSD-based forces, where much larger vectors can occur. Consequently, a smaller τ has to be chosen, which also impacts the amount of regularization. A pragmatic solution is to scale the update field to a maximal size, as discussed for example in [Kabus 2006].

Passive forces are defined based on the gradients of the reference image, which entails a computational advantage: The gradients remain fixed and therefore have to be computed only once. However, this can turn out to be disadvantageous with regard to accuracy. If a gradient points in the false direction – for example, due to noise or image artifacts in clinical data – the same incorrect force will be added in each iteration, only varying in magnitude but not in direction. This fault is only corrected by regularization. Active forces in contrast change in each iteration based on the transformed template image.

Another point worth of discussion is the convergence to a steady state solution. To terminate the registration, a stop criterion has to be defined that evaluates the progress of the algorithm. In this context, two aspects are of interest: a metric $\mathcal{M}$ that quantifies the quality of the computed transformation (similar to but not restricted to the energy (3.2)) and a criterion that constitutes if convergence is achieved given a certain number of subsequent values $\mathcal{M}^{(k)}$ for the most recent iterations. This aspect will be discussed in Chapter 7.

Chapter 4

Variational level set segmentation

The primary objective of this work is the consideration of knowledge about the patient's anatomy in registration algorithms to model morphological and physiological characteristics. Such knowledge can be provided by a segmentation of the organ or structure of interest. The focus of this chapter is therefore the presentation of a segmentation framework that can be combined with the registration model introduced in Chapter 3. Keeping this in mind, segmentation with level sets is particularly eligible because it can be formulated as an energy minimization problem. Equivalently to the registration framework, this allows not only a problem-specific adaption of the general segmentation approach, but also an intrinsic integration of segmentation and registration as presented in Chapter 5.

The basic framework for region-based level set segmentation is introduced in Section 4.1. Thereafter, some examples for problem-oriented formulation of specific energy terms are summarized (Section 4.2). Subsequently, an extension to multi-object segmentation is detailed (Section 4.3) and the framework is discussed in the concluding Section 4.4. Each section includes experiments using synthetic images to demonstrate the algorithms functionality.

4.1 Region-based level set segmentation

Deformable models are a commonly used approach to image segmentation. The underlying idea is a two-step procedure: First, an initial object boundary (for example a contour in 2D or a surface in 3D) is defined in the image. Then, this initialization is iteratively deformed until it traces the object borders depicted in the image. The fundamental property of a deformable model is the representation of the boundary, which ranges from discrete models like simplex meshes [Delingette 1999] or mass-spring models [Vasilescu and Terzopoulos 1992] to mathematically formulated active contours [Kass et al. 1987] and – as regarded in this work – level curves of higher-dimensional functions called *level sets*. Front propagation with level sets was first proposed by Osher and Sethian [1988] and applied to image segmentation by Caselles et al. [1993] and Malladi et al. [1995]. Later, Caselles et al. [1997] formulated the approach as

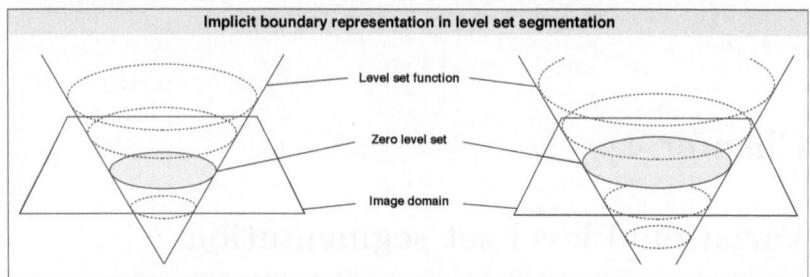

Figure 4.1: In level set segmentation, the object boundaries are implicitly formulated as the zero level curve of a higher-dimensional function, the so-called level set function ϕ. A deformation of the level set function implies a propagation of the object boundary.

an energy minimization problem and Chan and Vese [2001] extended it to region-based segmentation, which establishes the basis for the formulation presented in this chapter.

In level set segmentation, the object boundary is implicitly embedded as a level curve in a higher-dimensional function ϕ, the so-called level set function. This view can be compared to isopleths in geography or isobars in meteorology. From a mathematical point of view, let $\Sigma \subseteq \Omega$ be an open set describing the object in the image domain $\Omega \subset \mathbb{R}^d$. Its boundary $\Gamma := \partial\Sigma$ is embedded in the level set function $\phi : \Omega \to \mathbb{R}$ with

$$
\phi(\boldsymbol{x}) \begin{cases} < 0 & \text{if } \boldsymbol{x} \in \Sigma \\ > 0 & \text{if } \boldsymbol{x} \in \Omega \setminus \overline{\Sigma} \\ = 0 & \text{if } \boldsymbol{x} \in \Gamma \end{cases}
$$

as the zero level curve, the so-called zero level set $\Gamma = \{\boldsymbol{x} : \phi(\boldsymbol{x}) = 0\}$. Here, $\overline{\Sigma} = \Sigma \cup \partial\Sigma$ denotes the closure of the set. As illustrated in Figure 4.1, ϕ is usually defined to be a signed distance function $\phi(\boldsymbol{x}) := \mathrm{dist}(\boldsymbol{x}, \Gamma)$, where $\mathrm{dist}(\boldsymbol{x}, \Gamma)$ denotes the Euclidean distance of $\boldsymbol{x}$ to the closest point of Γ.

This representation brings several advantages. In contrast to explicitly formulated active contours, no re-parametrization of the level set function is required during the iteration process. Moreover, topological changes of the object are handled in a natural way. The method is also applicable to segment objects of arbitrary dimensions.

In correspondence to the registration problem presented in Chapter 3, an energy is defined that quantifies how well a level set function specifies the object in an image $I : \Omega \to \mathbb{R}$. The optimal function $\hat{\phi}$ is then determined by solving

$$
\hat{\phi} = \arg\min_{\phi} \mathcal{J}^{Seg}[\phi] , \tag{4.1}
$$

with

$$\mathcal{J}^{Seg}[\phi] := \mathcal{E}[I; \phi] + \alpha \mathcal{I}[\phi] \tag{4.2}$$

denoting the energy functional [Chan and Vese 2001]. Here, $\mathcal{E}$ denotes the external energy that measures how well the zero level set of ϕ separates the object from the background in the image. The internal energy $\mathcal{I}$ is appended to favor smooth objects and $\alpha \in \mathbb{R}^+$ is a weighting parameter.

4.1.1 Internal and external energy terms

To formulate specific energy terms, the Heaviside step function $H : \mathbb{R} \to [0, 1]$, defined in the sense of a distribution by

$$H(x) := \begin{cases} 0 & \text{if } x < 0 \\ 1 & \text{if } x \geq 0 \end{cases},$$

is used to describe inside and outside the object. Equivalently, the zero level set can be determined using the Dirac delta distribution $\delta : \mathbb{R} \to [0, \infty]$ with

$$\delta(x) := \begin{cases} 0 & \text{if } x \neq 0 \\ \infty & \text{if } x = 0 \end{cases}$$

and $\int_{-\infty}^{\infty} \delta(x) \, dx = 1$ (see Figure 4.2 for an illustration). This allows the internal energy to be defined as the length of the zero level set

$$\mathcal{I}[\phi] := \int_{\Omega} \|\nabla H(\phi(\boldsymbol{x}))\| \, d\boldsymbol{x} = \int_{\Omega} \delta(\phi(\boldsymbol{x})) \, \|\nabla \phi(\boldsymbol{x})\| \, d\boldsymbol{x} \,. \tag{4.3}$$

Minimizing this energy favors short contours and therefore results in a smoothing of the boundary.

Chan and Vese [2001] proposed the external energy

$$\mathcal{E}[I; \phi] := \int_{\Sigma} \left(\bar{I}_{in} - I(\boldsymbol{x})\right)^2 d\boldsymbol{x} + \int_{\Omega \setminus \Sigma} \left(\bar{I}_{out} - I(\boldsymbol{x})\right)^2 d\boldsymbol{x}$$
$$= \int_{\Omega} (1 - H(\phi(\boldsymbol{x}))) \left(\bar{I}_{in} - I(\boldsymbol{x})\right)^2 + H(\phi(\boldsymbol{x})) \left(\bar{I}_{out} - I(\boldsymbol{x})\right)^2 d\boldsymbol{x} \,,$$

where $\bar{I}_{in}$ and $\bar{I}_{out}$ denote the mean greyvalue inside and outside the object, respectively. This model is usually not versatile enough in clinical applications where object or background are composed of different structures with complex greyvalue distributions. Therefore, the more general formulation

$$\mathcal{E}[I; \phi] := - \int_{\Omega} (1 - H(\phi(\boldsymbol{x}))) \, \log p_{in}(I(\boldsymbol{x})) + H(\phi(\boldsymbol{x})) \, \log p_{out}(I(\boldsymbol{x})) \, d\boldsymbol{x} \,, \tag{4.4}$$

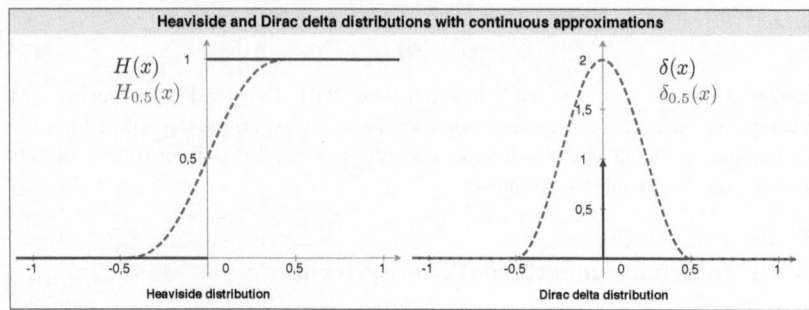

Figure 4.2: The Heaviside and Dirac delta distribution, which are used to formulate inside/outside and boundary of the object, respectively. Moreover, the continuous approximations used to obtain differentiability are illustrated.

is commonly utilized, where p_{in} and p_{out} denote the probability density functions for greyvalues inside and outside the object [Cremers et al. 2007; Schmidt-Richberg et al. 2009c]. The estimation of these functions – often using a training data set – is application-specific and will be discussed in Section 7.3.1.

4.1.2 Numerical solution

In correspondence to the registration approach presented in Chapter 3, the minimization problem (4.1) is solved using the calculus of variations. First, following Chan and Vese [2001], Heaviside and Dirac delta distributions are approximated using the continuous formulations

$$H_\epsilon(x) := \begin{cases} 1 & \text{if } x > \epsilon \\ 0 & \text{if } x < -\epsilon \\ \frac{1}{2}\left(1 + \frac{x}{\epsilon} + \frac{1}{\pi}\sin\left(\frac{\pi}{\epsilon}x\right)\right) & \text{if } |x| \leq \epsilon \end{cases}$$

and

$$\delta_\epsilon(x) := \frac{d}{dx}H_\epsilon(x) = \begin{cases} 0 & \text{if } |x| > \epsilon \\ \frac{1}{2\epsilon}\left(1 + \cos\left(\frac{\pi}{\epsilon}x\right)\right) & \text{if } |x| \leq \epsilon \end{cases}$$

to attain differentiability (see Figure 4.2). For convenience, the index ϵ is omitted in the following.

In accordance with Section 3.1.1, the Euler-Lagrange equation of the energy functional (4.2) is derived and a gradient descent is performed to find the minimum. With internal and external energy defined according to (4.3) and (4.4), the Euler-Lagrange equation for level set segmentation then reads

$$\partial_t\phi = -\delta(\phi)\left(-\log\frac{p_{out}}{p_{in}} - \alpha\nabla\frac{\nabla\phi}{\|\nabla\phi\|}\right). \tag{4.5}$$

The steps of the derivation are detailed in Appendix B.1.3. The corresponding explicit solution scheme is given by

$$\phi^{(k+1)} = \phi^{(k)} + \tau\delta(\phi^{(k)}) \left(\log \frac{p_{out}}{p_{in}} + \alpha\nabla \frac{\nabla\phi^{(k)}}{\|\nabla\phi^{(k)}\|} \right). \qquad (4.6)$$

4.1.3 Implementation

Complying with the solution scheme described by (4.6) implies that the complete level set function is updated in each iteration. In practice, however, only the region around the zero level set is of interest to describe the object boundary. Therefore, multiple approaches have been presented to restrain computation to this region, for example the narrow-band method [Adalsteinsson and Sethian 1994] and distance-regularized level sets [Li et al. 2010]. In this work, sparse field level sets following Whitaker [1998] are applied. Here, voxels x with $-0.5 \leq \phi(x) \leq 0.5$ – that means voxels that contain the object boundary – are considered to lie in the *active set* of voxels. Only the active set is updated each iteration according to (4.6). To compute the derivatives in $\nabla\phi$ via finite difference approximation, additionally d layers of neighboring voxels are updated such that ϕ maintains the characteristics of a distance function. For details on the algorithm, the reader is referred to [Whitaker 1998].

4.1.4 Experiments

In Figure 4.3, a simple example for level set segmentation is given. The contour slowly propagates outwards until the boundary of the object is reached in the image. The propagation process is steered by the greyvalue probability distributions p_{in} and p_{out}, which in this example are modeled by Gaussian distributions around the mean greyvalues inside and outside, respectively.

The second experiment shown in Figure 4.4 illustrates the influence of the curvature weight α. If it is chosen small ($\alpha = 1$), the level set propagates into each of the thin structures in the image, except the one only one pixel wide. If the curvature weight is increased, small structures are omitted by the segmentation. A very high α even results in a segmentation of background regions in favor of a smooth object boundary.

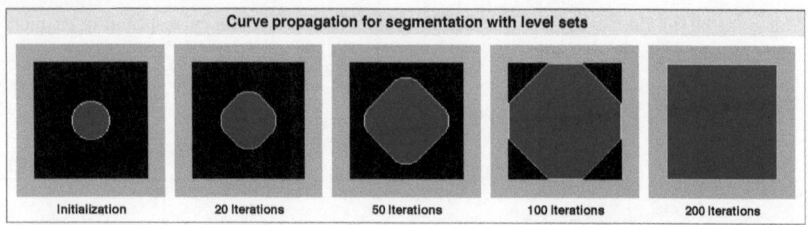

Figure 4.3: A simple example for level set segmentation on the course of 200 iterations ($\tau = 0.5$, $\alpha = 1.0$).

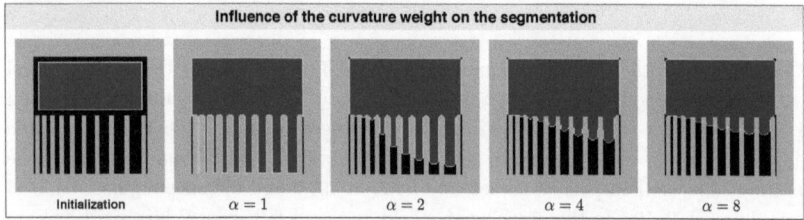

Figure 4.4: Segmentation of an object with thin structures with different choices of the curvature weight α (200 iterations, $\tau = 0.5$).

4.2 Extended energy terms for problem-specific modeling

The basic framework presented in the previous section can be extended in various ways for a problem-specific adaption of the algorithm. For example, Forkert et al. [2012] define an energy based on the vesselness filter to steer propagation into small vessel structures for vessel segmentation in brain MRI images. Prior information about typical shape and shape variations of the object is integrated in the form of a statistical shape model (SSM) into the level set framework by Hufnagel et al. [2009]. Cremers et al. [2007] propose a probabilistic combination with manually defined user labels, aiming for an interactive optimization of segmentation results.

These examples represent only a fraction of possible modeling approaches. However, instead of giving a comprehensive overview on current methods, the focus of this section lies on the presentation of two particular extensions that will be of interest in following chapters: a segmentation refinement based on a prior shape (Section 4.2.1) and an edge-based stopping term (Section 4.2.2).

4.2.1 Prior shape information for segmentation refinement

In some applications, coarse segmentations are available that lack accuracy and/or smoothness. Such estimates can origin from basic image processing steps (for example a region growing with subsequent morphological operations), an atlas segmentation transferred to the image using image registration techniques, or a manual segmentation process. In particular in the latter case, a slice-by-slice segmentation of the object by a clinical expert often results in an insufficiently smooth boundary, especially in z-direction. This effect is aggravated by imaging and reconstruction artifacts in the data.

To circumvent this problem, a level set-based refinement of the segmentation can be performed. With this goal, the given coarse segmentation serves on the one hand as initialization, on the other hand as prior shape information for the segmentation process: While small derivations from this shape are possible – aiming for example for a smoother surface and a more accurate tracing of the object boundaries – the zero level set is restrained from propagating substantially apart.

From a mathematical perspective, let $\tilde{\phi}(\boldsymbol{x})$ be the level set function corresponding to a coarse segmentation resulting from any manual or (semi-)automatic segmentation process. An improved segmentation $\phi(\boldsymbol{x})$ is computed by minimizing the energy functional

$$\mathcal{J}^{Seg}[\phi] := \mathcal{E}[I; \phi] + \alpha \mathcal{I}[\phi] + \beta \mathcal{P}[\tilde{\phi}; \phi].$$

Exploiting the fact that the value of the level set function at a point $\boldsymbol{x}$ specifies the distance of this point to the object boundary, the third energy term

$$\mathcal{P}[\tilde{\phi}; \phi] := \frac{1}{2} \int_{\Omega} \delta(\phi(\boldsymbol{x})) \left(\tilde{\phi}(\boldsymbol{x}) - \phi(\boldsymbol{x})\right)^2 d\boldsymbol{x} \qquad (4.7)$$

acts as a prior shape term for the segmentation by penalizing large derivations of ϕ from $\tilde{\phi}$. The parameter $\beta \in \mathbb{R}^+$ weights the influence of the prior segmentation. After some simplifications detailed in Appendix B.1.3.3, the gradient descent scheme (4.5) with additional prior shape information reads

$$\partial_t \phi = -\delta(\phi) \left(-\log \frac{p_{out}}{p_{in}} - \alpha \nabla \frac{\nabla \phi}{\|\nabla \phi\|} - \beta(\tilde{\phi} - \phi)\right).$$

4.2.2 Edge attraction terms

Several formulations exist for edge-based level sets, most prominent the *Geodesic Active Contours* introduced by Caselles et al. [1997]. However, these formulations are not compatible with the framework presented in Section 4.1 in a straightforward manner. Therefore, a slightly different formulation is used in this work.

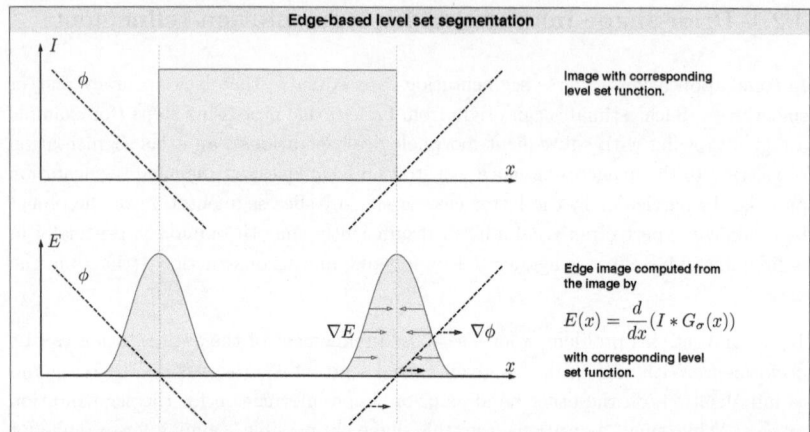

Figure 4.5: Definition of the edge-based energy term by the assumption that gradients $\nabla\phi$ of the level set function and ∇E of the edge image point in the same directions inside the object and in opposite directions outside the object.

In a first step, an edge map $E : \Omega \to \mathbb{R}$ is computed from I by

$$E := \left\| \nabla(I * G_\sigma) \right\|,$$

where G_σ denotes a Gaussian filter kernel with standard deviation σ. As illustrated in Figure 4.5, a correct segmentation implies that the gradients of edge image E and level set function ϕ point in the same direction inside the object (that means, $\nabla\phi \cdot \nabla E$ is positive) and in opposite directions outside ($\nabla\phi \cdot \nabla E$ negative). This observation leads to the energy formulation

$$\mathcal{G}[E; \phi] := \frac{1}{2} \int_\Omega H(\phi(\boldsymbol{x}))\nabla\phi(\boldsymbol{x}) \cdot \nabla E(\boldsymbol{x}) - \left(1 - H(\phi(\boldsymbol{x}))\right)\nabla\phi(\boldsymbol{x}) \cdot \nabla E(\boldsymbol{x}) \, d\boldsymbol{x}$$
$$= \int_\Omega \left(H(\phi(\boldsymbol{x})) - 0.5\right)\nabla\phi(\boldsymbol{x}) \cdot \nabla E(\boldsymbol{x}) \, d\boldsymbol{x}, \tag{4.8}$$

which can be applied either instead of or in addition to the region-based external energy $\mathcal{E}$. A derivation of the Euler Lagrange equation (see Appendix B.1.3.4) leads to the gradient descent scheme

$$\partial_t\phi = -\delta(\phi)\left(-\log\frac{p_{out}}{p_{in}} - \alpha\nabla\frac{\nabla\phi}{\|\nabla\phi\|} + \gamma\nabla\phi \cdot \nabla E\right) \tag{4.9}$$

for a combined edge- and region-based segmentation, where $\gamma \in \mathbb{R}^+$ is a positive weighting parameter.

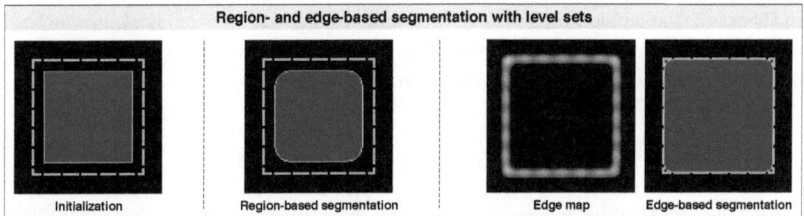

Figure 4.6: Experiment demonstrating the situational benefit of edge-based segmentation (100 iterations, $\alpha = 1.0$, $\tau = 0.5$). Since the greyvalue distributions inside and outside the object are not distinguishable, the region-based term fails in this example.

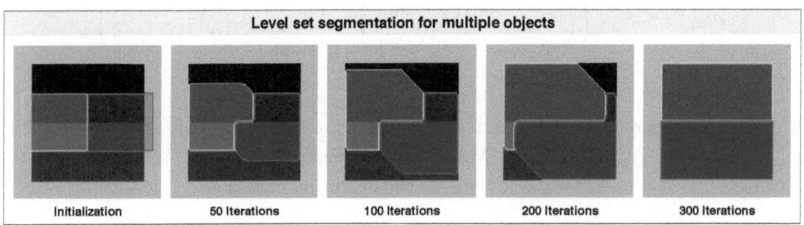

Figure 4.7: Simultaneous segmentation of three objects including the background, which is not visualized as color overly ($\alpha = 1.0$, $\tau = 0.5$). Each object has a greyvalue distribution distinguishable from the other objects.

4.2.3 Experiments

The purpose of edge-based level set segmentation is illustrated in Figure 4.6. In this example, object and background have the same greyvalue distributions and are only delimited by a low-contrasted edge in the image. Region-based segmentation fails because $p_{in} = p_{out}$, such that only a smoothing of the level set function is performed. If the image is smoothed instead and interpreted as an edge map, the object boundaries are traced correctly by the algorithm presented in Section 4.2.2.

4.3 Level sets with multiple objects

Using the framework described in Sections 4.1 and 4.2, a single object can be separated from the background. To simultaneously segment multiple objects – for example the five pulmonary lobes – the level set framework has to be extended in this matter. Several approaches have been proposed for this purpose, in most of which a level set function is employed for each object and a coupling force is defined to avoid gaps or overlapping of the objects [Zhao et al. 1996; Samson et al. 1999; Paragios and Deriche 2000].

In this work, the method proposed by Brox and Weickert [2004] is followed, in which no additional force is required. The approach is based on the observation that the gradient descent scheme (4.5) can be reformulated to

$$\partial_t \phi = -\delta(\phi) \left(\left(\log p_{in} - \frac{\alpha}{2} \nabla \frac{\nabla \phi}{\|\nabla \phi\|} \right) - \left(\log p_{out} - \frac{\alpha}{2} \nabla \frac{\nabla(-\phi)}{\|\nabla(-\phi)\|} \right) \right).$$

Envisioning two complementary level set functions $\phi_{in} := \phi$ and $\phi_{out} := -\phi$ of object and background, this formulation can be interpreted as a competition of object- and background-related forces:

$$\partial_t \phi_{in} = -\delta(\phi) \left(\left(\log p_{in} - \frac{\alpha}{2} \nabla \frac{\nabla \phi_{in}}{\|\nabla \phi_{in}\|} \right) - \left(\log p_{out} - \frac{\alpha}{2} \nabla \frac{\nabla \phi_{out}}{\|\nabla \phi_{out}\|} \right) \right)$$

$$=: -\delta(\phi) \left(f_{in} - f_{out} \right).$$

This idea is extended to N competing functions ϕ_i, $i = 0, \ldots, N-1$, each representing one object $\Sigma_i := \{ \boldsymbol{x} : \phi_i(\boldsymbol{x}) < 0 \}$. Minimizing the energy functional (4.2) under the constraints $\bigcap_i \Sigma_i = \emptyset$ and $\bigcup_i \Sigma_i = \Omega$ leads to the evolution equation

$$\partial_t \phi_i = -\delta(\phi_i) \left(f_i - \max_{H(\phi_j) < 0, j \neq i} (f_j, f_i - 1) \right) \quad \text{with} \quad f_k := \log p_k - \frac{\alpha}{2} \nabla \frac{\nabla \phi_k}{\|\nabla \phi_k\|}. \quad (4.10)$$

In this formulation, the (mostly outwards-directed) force f_i, which affects to the level set ϕ_i, competes with the maximal force of all adhering level set functions ϕ_j. The additional term $f_i - 1$ balances the force if no other object is in the proximity.

4.3.1 Experiments

The simultaneous segmentation of multiple objects is demonstrated in Figure 4.7. Note that three level set functions are employed: one each for upper and lower part of the object and one for the background. An individual greyvalue distributions p_k can be assigned to each of these objects, which enables a correct segmentation of the three regions.

4.4 Discussion

In this chapter, a segmentation method using level sets was introduced. In particular, the flexibility of the approach was highlighted by summarizing several possibilities for an extension of the model aiming for a problem-specific adaption.

Two prerequisites are required by the algorithm to obtain satisfying results. First, adequate probability distribution have to be given to differentiate between objects. This also reveals a major drawback of the method, which is not applicable for texture-based differentiation between objects if the probability density functions of different textures are alike. Second, segmentation success often depends on a reasonably good initialization of the level set function. This is even more true for edge-based segmentation terms to avoid that the zero level set is attracted by neighboring structures.

From a mathematical point of view, the segmentation model is formulated as an energy minimization problem and solved using the calculus of variations. Due to this, it is possible to reconcile the segmentation approach with the registration framework presented in Chapter 6 in a straightforward manner. This will be in the focus of the following Chapter 5.

It should be noted that – strictly speaking – the extended approach for multi-object segmentation presented in Section 4.3 no longer solves the minimization problem (4.1). This is due to the formulation with the max function in (4.10).

Chapter 5

Lung registration with explicit interlobular fissure alignment

The human lungs consist of five separate lobes, three in the right lung and two in the left. The lobes have individual bronchial and vascular systems and are functioning relatively independent from each other. Moreover, each lobe has its own pleural covering. As illustrated in Figure 5.1, the pleurae of adhering lobes are visible as hairlines in radiographic images and are denoted as the interlobular fissures [Hayashi et al. 2001].

In lung registration, a precise alignment of the fissures indicates correctly established correspondences between the individual lobes. However, while algorithms for lung registration generally exhibit a high accuracy, results also often show an insufficient alignment of the lung fissures. Due to anatomical divergences, this problem is particularly severe for inter-patient registration, but it is also evident for intra-patient registration and motion estimation. For example, Murphy et al. [2011b] state for the EMPIRE10 study that while *"most of the algorithms performed extremely well in terms of both singularities and lung boundary alignment, [...] differences are much more apparent in the fissure alignment category."*

Deficient fissure alignment has mainly two reasons: First, fissures are mostly depicted with very low contrast – especially in low-dose CT images – and intensity-based

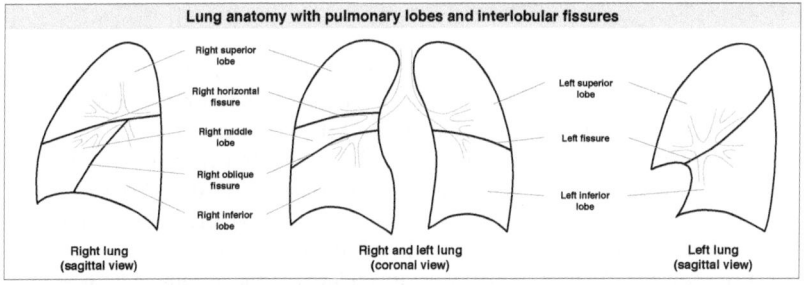

Figure 5.1: Anatomy of the lung and the pulmonary lobes.

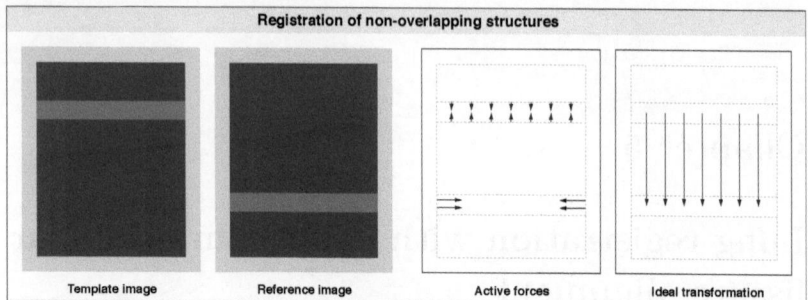

Figure 5.2: Illustration of the problem arising when matching the low-contrasted structure (idealized fissures) in template and reference image using a classical intensity-based registration approach: Since the structures are not overlapping, forces as shown in the third image are generated – in the example active forces, see Section 3.2; the last image shows the intended deformation.

registration is therefore difficult. There are also few vessels in the proximity of fissures, which leads to homogeneous greyvalues in this region. Second, to steer iterative algorithms in the right direction, structures usually have to be overlapping (see Figure 5.2). While multi-scale approaches and regularization schemes implicitly address these problems, small structures such as the fissures are not visible on coarse scales and no forces are explicitly generated that align disjunct structures as caused by large displacements or anatomical dissimilarities.

Few approaches have been published that directly address fissure alignment in registration. Van Rikxoort et al. [2010] combine a fissure enhancement filtering (cf. Section 5.2) and fissure locations approximated by airway segmentations to estimate distance maps to the fissures. These are then integrated in a registration approach, but image intensities are not considered. Related but not targeted at fissure alignment is the work of Cao et al. [2010a]. Here, the vesselness filter presented by Frangi et al. [1998] is used to define an additional registration term – called Sum of Squared Vesselness Measure Difference (SSVMD) – with the aim of aligning blood vessels.

Inspired by these ideas, an alternative approach is pursued in this work. Here, the problem of fissure alignment is addressed by integrating morphological knowledge about the lobes into the registration algorithm. This is achieved by combining a shape-based lobe segmentation approach with the intensity-based registration framework. For this purpose, the registration and segmentation approaches presented in Chapter 3 and 4, respectively, are first combined to a joint framework (Section 5.1). In Section 5.2, the basic level set segmentation is than extended for the specific task of lobe segmentation in CT images. Finally, lobe segmentation is employed in the integrated framework in Section 5.3 aiming for improved fissure alignment.

5.1 Combining registration and segmentation

Apart from the registration of clinical image data, the segmentation of anatomical objects in images is a major challenges in medical image processing. Consequently, numerous methods for either of these tasks have been developed in the past. In recent years, however, registration and segmentation techniques have increasingly been combined to joint approaches, which aim at exploiting the mutual dependency between both problems: For example, the knowledge about corresponding objects in reference and template image can improve the registration. Vice versa, correspondences between two images established by registration can be used to guide a segmentation algorithm.

In this section, a framework for integrated segmentation and registration is presented, which unites the variational non-linear registration and level set segmentation introduced in Chapter 3 and Chapter 4, respectively. First, in Section 5.1.1, an overview on current approaches for this purpose is given. A variational framework for joint registration and segmentation is then presented in Section 5.1.2.

5.1.1 Current methods for integrated registration and segmentation

Various approaches for simultaneous registration and segmentation have been published in the past. The most distinctive characteristics are represented by the transformation model and the formulation of the object in the segmentation component.

In statistical approaches, pixel-based segmentation with Markov Random Fields [Wyatt and Noble 2003] or Gibbs probability distributions [Flach and Schlesinger 2002] is combined with a registration based on rigid or affine transformations. Due to the computational complexity, only 2D images are regarded in these references. Pohl et al. [2006] propose an expectation maximization (EM) algorithm for joint classification and registration of a brain atlas with patient data using a composite global and object-specific transformation. For the same purpose, a more complex transformation modeled defined by a linear combination of about a thousand cosine transform bases is employed in [Ashburner and Friston 2005]. Such probabilistic approaches cannot be easily reconciled with the variational setting followed in this work and are therefore not further regarded.

However, several approaches exist that aim at combining registration and segmentation by minimization of a joint energy functional. Active contour segmentation and affine registration are combined in [Yezzi et al. 2003] using 2D images. A similar method for the correction of rigid rotation and translation in MR image series is proposed by Song et al. [2006]. An et al. [2005] add a non-linear deformation component defined at the contour points. A joint approach to propagate active contour segmentations through the slices of a volume image was presented by Young and Levy [2005]. More recently, Droske and Rumpf [2007] proposed a method for joint segmentation, registration and image denoising. Here, segmentation is carried out by the computation of the phase field function, which depends on a set of edges in the image.

Level sets are for example applied by Paragios [2003] for a simultaneous segmentation and tracking of the left ventricular myocardium. The underlying transformation can be either parametric (rigid, affine) or described by a local deformation field at the object surface. A similar approach is followed by Unal and Slabaugh [2005]. With application to radiation therapy, Lu et al. [2011] combine level set segmentation with registration based on free-form deformation (FFD) to align the planning CT/MR with a cone-beam CT/MR (CBCT/MR) assessed at treatment day. In [Ens et al. 2008], a dense elastic registration with Mutual Information as distance measure is combined with level set segmentation. The method presented in this chapter is based on [Schmidt-Richberg et al. 2008, 2009c] and combines level-set segmentation and non-linear registration in a variational framework.

5.1.2 A variational model for integrated registration and segmentation

The principle idea of the method introduced in [Schmidt-Richberg et al. 2009c] is illustrated in Figure 5.3. A baseline image B with corresponding segmentation of the structure of interest ϕ_B is assumed to be known in the process. This image can either be a mean intensity atlas created from an image pool, a segmented scan of a different patient or a particular time point in a follow-up study or 4D data set. A segmentation of an examined image I can be obtained on two ways: on the one hand, by direct (level set) segmentation of the structure (see Chapter 4); on the other hand, by registration of baseline and examined image – for example, using the method presented Chapter 3 – and a subsequent transformation of the baseline segmentation to the domain of I using the computed transformation φ. Ideally, the segmentations ϕ_I and $\phi_B \circ \varphi$ obtained in this way are identical. This evidence is exploited to couple registration and segmentation: By additionally demanding that both segmentations are similar to each other, consistent results of both methods are favored.

Referring to the formulations in Chapter 3 and Chapter 4, the integrated registration and segmentation model is formulated as a minimization problem. That means, a segmentation ϕ_I and a transformation φ are computed by minimizing the joint energy functional

$$\mathcal{J}^{Joint}[\varphi, \phi_I] := \mathcal{J}^{Reg}[\varphi] + \beta \mathcal{J}^{Seg}[\phi_I] + \beta_1 \mathcal{P}[\phi_B; \varphi, \phi_I]\,. \tag{5.1}$$

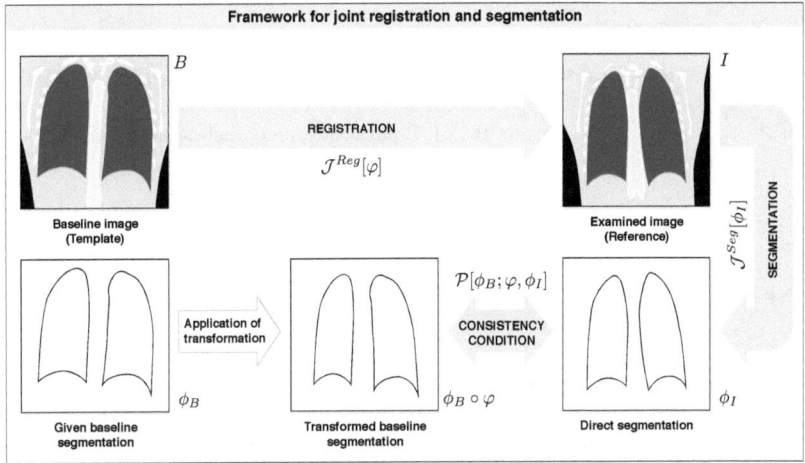

Figure 5.3: Illustration of the presented approach for joint registration and segmentation. A baseline image B with a corresponding segmentation ϕ_B is assumed to be given. A segmentation of an image of interest I is obtained on the one hand by direct level set segmentation, on the other hand by registration of B and I and subsequent transformation of ϕ_B to the domain of I. An additional condition demands similarity between ϕ_I and $\phi_B \circ \varphi$ and thereby connects registration and segmentation.

Here, registration and segmentation components are defined by (3.2) and (4.2), respectively. The constants $\beta, \beta_1 \in \mathbb{R}^+$ weight the terms against each other. In addition, the consistency condition

$$\mathcal{P}[\phi_B; \varphi, \phi_I] := \frac{1}{2} \int_\Omega \delta(\phi_I) \left(\phi_B \circ \varphi - \phi_I\right)^2 \, d\boldsymbol{x}$$

is defined based on the shape prior term (4.7), except that the coarse (manual) segmentation $\widetilde{\phi}$ is replaced by the transformed baseline segmentation $\phi_B \circ \varphi$. In detail, large distances between the zero level set of ϕ_I and the transformed baseline segmentation $\phi_B \circ \varphi$ are penalized, exploiting the fact that the value of a level set function is defined to be the distance to the closest boundary (cf. Section 4.2.1). This term therefore prevents the segmentation from markedly diverging from the transformed baseline segmentation and thus establishes the connection between the registration and segmentation components.

Without loss of generality, the transformation is defined in this section by a dense displacement field via $\varphi(\boldsymbol{x}) := \boldsymbol{x} - \boldsymbol{u}(\boldsymbol{x})$. The functional (5.1) is then alternately minimized in direction of $\boldsymbol{u}$ and ϕ_I. In detail, first ϕ_I is assumed to be constant and the Euler-Lagrange equation is derived for $\boldsymbol{u}$ as variable. This leads to the gradient descent scheme

$$\partial_t \boldsymbol{u} = -\boldsymbol{f}(\boldsymbol{u}) + \alpha_1 \mathcal{A}\boldsymbol{u} + \beta_1 \delta(\phi_I)\Big(\phi_B \circ \varphi - \phi_I\Big)\nabla(\phi_B \circ \varphi)\,, \tag{5.2}$$

for the registration (see Appendix B.1.4). Equivalently, an optimization in the direction of ϕ_I yields

$$\partial_t \phi_I = -\delta(\phi_I)\left(-\frac{\log p_{out}}{\log p_{in}} - \alpha_2 \nabla \frac{\nabla \phi_I}{\|\nabla \phi_I\|} - \beta_2(\phi_B \circ \varphi - \phi_I)\right) \tag{5.3}$$

with $\beta_2 := \beta_1/\beta$.

5.1.3 Numerical solution

Solution schemes for (5.2) and (5.3) are derived by a discretization of time in correspondence to (3.8) and (4.6), respectively. Doing so introduces two step sizes τ_1 for the registration and τ_2 for the segmentation.

Since the segmentation converges faster than the registration, a small value has to be chosen for β in (5.1) to balance both components. However, this implies a slow convergence of the approach. Therefore, multiple ($L \in \mathbb{N}$ with $L > 1$) registration iterations are instead performed for each segmentation iteration. The final algorithm is summarized in Algorithm 5.1.

Algorithm 5.1 Joint registration and segmentation.

Set $k = 0$, $\vec{U}^{(0)}$ to zero and let $\vec{\phi}_I^{(0)} \leftarrow \vec{\phi}_B$.
repeat
    Compute segmentation step.   ▷ Equation (5.3)
    Compute transformed segmentation $(\phi_B(\varphi^{(k)}(\boldsymbol{x}_j)))_{j=1,\dots,N}$.
    for $l = 1 \to L$ **do**
        Compute registration step.   ▷ Equation (5.2)
    end for
    Let $k \leftarrow k + 1$.
until algorithm converges or $k = k_{max}$.

5.1.4 Experiments

To demonstrate the functionality of the joint registration and segmentation framework, the synthetic example shown in Figure 5.4 is regarded. This is particularly challenging due to topology changes between baseline (template) and examined (reference) image. The ideal transformation is therefore not continuous between the objects and it is impossible to obtain the reference image by a transformation of the template image.

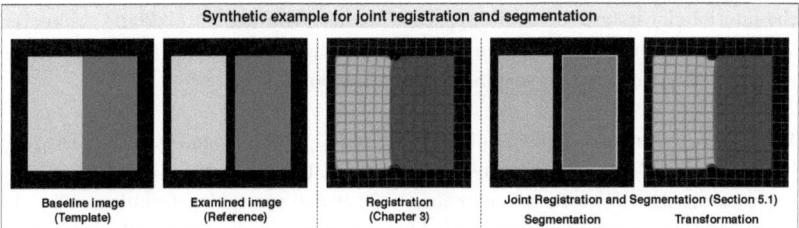

Figure 5.4: In this example, a correct alignment of both objects is impossible due to the change of topology. As a consequence, only he light object is correctly aligned since this is energetically favorable (center image). By integrating a segmentation of the dark structure and minimizing (5.1), a correct alignment of this object can be achieved. Experiments were performed using semi-implicit diffusion registration with active forces and $\tau_1 = 0.5$, $\alpha_1 = 1.0$, $\beta_1 = 0.25$, $\tau_2 = 0.5$, $\alpha_2 = 0.5$, $\beta_2 = 0.1$ and 1000 iterations on one level.

The intrinsic behavior of the algorithm is to match the light structure as good as possible because it exhibits the higher contrast with the background, that means a misalignment is less favorable in terms of energy minimization. As a consequence, the darker structure is falsely deformed. Applying the joint segmentation and registration approach presented in this section, the registration can be influenced to focus on a correct alignment of the darker object at the expense of the lighter object.

5.2 Pulmonary lobe segmentation using level sets

To employ the presented joint registration and segmentation framework with the aim of improved fissure alignment, the segmentation component is required to be suitable for pulmonary lobe segmentation. This is not provided by the basic level set formulation introduced in Section 4.1. Therefore, an application-specific extension of this approach is presented in the following, aiming at a simultaneous segmentation of the lung and the pulmonary lobes in thoracic CT images.

Below, an overview on current methods for lung and lobe segmentation is given (Section 5.2.1). Based on [Schmidt-Richberg et al. 2012d], a novel level set-based approach is subsequently presented in Section 5.2.2. Its principle functionality is demonstrated using synthetic images in Section 5.2.3.

5.2.1 Current methods for lung and lobe segmentation

A robust segmentation of the lung and the individual lobes is required for many applications in computer aided diagnostics and intervention. For example, it is clinically important to determine if affections in early stages are confined to single lobes, since the interlobular fissures stem the spread of diseases [Hayashi et al. 2001]. Moreover, accurate segmentations are required to characterize and quantify malfunctions like residual pulmonary parenchyma [Sluimer et al. 2006].

Lung segmentation   Many applicable techniques for the segmentation of the lung boundaries in CT images have been proposed in the past. Since the lung is well-contrasted with the surrounding tissue, basic image processing techniques like the region-growing algorithm induce reasonable results. Therefore, most publications rather focus on post-processing and improving the algorithms' robustness. For example, Hu et al. [2001] first used an optimal thresholding with a subsequent connectivity analysis for lung segmentation. Furthermore, a morphological closing of inner lung cavities, an automatic removal of trachea and main airways and a specific smoothing technique were deployed to improve the results. Van Rikxoort et al. [2009] extended the approach to automatically detect errors that can be caused for example by pathologies. Error detection was realized by considering lung volume plausibility and shape consistency. A multi-atlas approach was used for correction. Messay et al. [2010] further proposed a subsequent segmentation refinement process using a rolling ball filter. A 4D statistical shape model is used by Wilms et al. [2012] to simultaneously segment all time points of a 4D data set.

Lobe segmentation   In contrast to lung segmentation, a segmentation of the lobes is generally considered to be a very challenging task if the images lack in quality or if anatomical anomalies occur. Therefore and due to its clinical relevance, a wide variety of approaches has been proposed. Most methods start from a segmentation of the interlobular fissures to separate the lobes. Wang et al. [2006] propose a curve-growing process based on image features and atlas information to segment the fissures. Among others, Wiemker et al. [2005] and Lassen et al. [2010] proposed a fissure enhancement based on the eigenvectors of the Hessian matrix, similar to the vesselness measure. Van Rikxoort et al. [2008] extended this approach to a supervised learning method based on the second order derivatives of the image.

Most of these techniques perform well if images are of reasonably good quality. However, a detection of the fissures is often not sufficient to separate the lobes because fissures are incomplete for many subjects due to anatomical conditions or severe lung diseases [Aziz et al. 2004]. Moreover, bad image quality and insufficient spatial resolution can cause fragmentary segmentations. This was addressed by Pu et al. [2009] using an implicit surface fitting with different radial basis functions. Van Rikxoort et al. [2010] instead proposed an atlas-based completion of the fissures. A sampling of fissure particles based on maximum a posteriori probabilities (MAP) of image features followed by a thin plate spline interpolation was used by Ross et al. [2010]. Zhang et al. [2006] applied a fuzzy decision system considering image and atlas information for lobe segmentation. Ukil and Reinhardt [2009] later applied Fast Marching Methods to complete fissures in projection images.

5.2.2 Extension of the region-based level set framework for lobe segmentation

The approach presented in this section is based on the techniques introduced in Sections 4.1 to 4.3. The air-containing lung features a greyvalue distribution well distinguishable from the background, which is composed of the ribs, the liver and other soft tissue. Therefore, the basic region-based segmentation approach (4.6) is applicable 'out of the box' given p_{in} and p_{out} and an initial segmentation.

To segment the five human lobes, $N = 6$ objects (background and five lobes) have to be employed using the multi-object approach presented in Section 4.3. Here, ϕ_0 is used for the background and ϕ_i with $i = 1, \ldots, 5$ for the five lobes in an arbitrary order. Since all lobes have (approximately) the same greyvalue distributions, $p_i := p_{in}$ and $p_0 := p_{out}$ is valid. Using the model described by (4.10) leads to a propagation of ϕ_0 in direction of the lung boundaries. However, since p_i equals p_j if $i, j \in \{1, \ldots, 5\}$, only a smoothing of the level set function is performed between two lobes. To this end, a cost image C is computed as the distance map to a fissure segmentation and incorporated in the segmentation model using the edge attraction term (4.9), such that it draws the contour to the interlobular fissures. This procedure is detailed in the following.

5.2.2.1 Fissure-attraction term for lobe segmentation

In the first step, the interlobular fissures are segmented using an automatic approach. This step is principally generic and the specific algorithm can be chosen freely. However, to prevent the level sets from being attracted by structures wrongly classified as fissures, it is advisable to aim at a high specificity at the expense of sensitivity. Therefore and following the evaluation study in [Schmidt-Richberg et al. 2012c], the automatic supervised enhancement filter proposed by van Rikxoort et al. [2008] is chosen in this work.

In CT images, fissures generally show little contrast to the surrounding lung tissue. Moreover, they are imaged with greyvalues very similar to those of bronchial and blood vessels (around -800 HU), which considerably aggravates an intensity-based differentiation between these structures. Therefore – in accordance with most other methods for fissure detection – van Rikxoort et al. [2008] proposed to additionally consider shape information by detecting two-dimensional (that means, planar) objects in three-dimensional space. From a mathematical perspective, the local shape of a structure at a point $\boldsymbol{x} \in \Omega$ can be assessed by considering the eigenvalues λ_0, λ_1 and λ_2 of the Hessian matrix $\mathcal{H}(I(\boldsymbol{x}))$ with $|\lambda_0| \geq |\lambda_1| \geq |\lambda_2|$. For plane-like structures, $|\lambda_0|$ is large (across plane) and $|\lambda_1|$ and $|\lambda_2|$ are small (in-plane).

Based on a set of training images with known fissure segmentations, the general idea of the algorithm is to sample intensity- and shape-based features at fissure- and non-fissure voxels and then train a statistical classifier to recognize the fissures in a test image. For this purpose, a set of 57 features was identified. In detail, these are the image greyvalue (1 feature) and – each computed on four different scales with smoothing weights $\sigma = 1, 2, 4, 8$ – the greyvalues of the smoothed images ($4 \cdot 1$ feature), the gradient components ($4 \cdot 3$), gradient magnitude ($4 \cdot 1$), the components of the Hessian matrix ($4 \cdot 6$) and its eigenvalues ($4 \cdot 3$). A subset these features (here: nine features) is chosen according to [van Rikxoort et al. 2008] and used to train a k-nearest neighbors ($k$nn) classifier with $k = 15$.

The classifier provides a fissureness image $F : \Omega \to \{0, \dots, k\}$, in which each voxel value indicates the number $m \leq k$ of the k nearest neighbors that were classified as fissure. The output of the first classification run is then used as input in a second run using 14 features as proposed by van Rikxoort et al. [2008]. This two-phase strategy significantly reduces the influence of background noise on the classification procedure. Again aiming for high specificity, the output of the second run is then thresholded at $m \geq 14$ and a morphological closing followed by a connected-component analysis is performed to exclude small structures caused by noise.

Finally, the goal is to define a cost image that is zero at the fissures and high in distant regions. It is therefore proceeded by computing the topological skeleton K of the fissure segmentation and defining the cost image $C : \Omega \to \mathbb{R}$ by $C(\boldsymbol{x}) := \sqrt{\text{dist}(\boldsymbol{x}, K)}$, where $\text{dist}(\boldsymbol{x}, K)$ is the Euclidean distance of point $\boldsymbol{x}$ to the closest point of the skeleton K. With this, the force term in (4.10) can be reformulated to incorporate a fissure-attraction force by

$$\partial_t \phi_i = -\delta(\phi_i) \left(f_i - \max_{H(\phi_j) < 0, j \neq i} (f_j, f_i - 1) \right)$$

with

$$f_k := \log p_k - \frac{\alpha}{2} \nabla \frac{\nabla \phi_k}{\|\nabla \phi_k\|} - \frac{\gamma}{2} \nabla \phi_k \cdot \nabla C \,, \tag{5.4}$$

where the last term corresponds to the gradient attraction term in (4.9).

5.2.3 Experiments

The simultaneous segmentation of lung and lung lobes is illustrated using the synthetic example shown in Figure 5.5. In contrast to Figure 4.7, the upper and lower part of the object simulating the pulmonary lobes do not feature different greyvalues and are only divided by a low-contrast edge, the idealized fissure. Accordingly, the standard multi-object segmentation as presented in Section 4.3 fails: While the outside boundary corresponding to the lung is segmented correctly, no force drives the object to the edge in the inside (compare Figure 4.6). Incorporating a cost image derived from a fissure segmentation as proposed in this section and considering intensity as well as shape information results in a correct segmentation of the two objects and the background.

An extensive evaluation study of the algorithm for lobe segmentation using clinical image data is given in Section 7.3.

5.3 Integrated registration with pulmonary lobe segmentation

In a final step, the problem of fissure alignment is addressed by using the joint registration and segmentation framework introduced in Section 5.1 in conjunction with the segmentation of the pulmonary lobes presented in Section 5.2. In detail, the lobe segmentation is integrated in the registration approach to generate forces that cause an explicit alignment of fissures and lung boundaries in baseline and examined image.

With this purpose, the prior shape term is extended for multiple regions to simultaneously deal with the five human lobes:

$$\mathcal{P}[\boldsymbol{\phi}_A; \varphi, \boldsymbol{\phi}_I] := \frac{1}{2N} \int_\Omega \sum_{i=0}^{N-1} \delta(\phi_{I,i}) \Big(\phi_{B,i} \circ \varphi - \phi_{I,i} \Big)^2 d\boldsymbol{x} \,,$$

with $N = 6$ and $\boldsymbol{\phi}_I = (\phi_{I,i})_{i=0,\dots,N-1}$ holding the segmentations of the objects in image I. Using this expression, the gradient descent of the registration is described by

$$\frac{\partial \varphi}{\partial t} = -\boldsymbol{f}(\boldsymbol{u}) + \alpha_1 \mathcal{A}\boldsymbol{u} + \frac{\beta_1}{N} \sum_{i=0}^{N-1} \delta(\phi_{I,i}) \Big(\phi_{B,i} \circ \varphi - \phi_{I,i} \Big) \nabla(\phi_{B,i} \circ \varphi) \,.$$

For the segmentation, the approach presented in Section 5.2 is applied 'out of the box' with additional inclusion of the prior shape term. This yields

$$f_k := \log p_k - \frac{\alpha_2}{2} \nabla \frac{\nabla \phi_{I,k}}{\|\nabla \phi_{I,k}\|} - \frac{\beta_2}{2} (\phi_{B,k} \circ \varphi - \phi_{I,k}) - \frac{\gamma}{2} \nabla \phi_{I,k} \cdot \nabla C$$

for the force computation following the multi-object segmentation scheme (4.10).

5.3.1 Experiments

In Figure 5.6 abstracted lungs with two lobes are shown. A standard registration of these image does not result in an alignment of the fissures. Instead, the transformation in the fissure region only causes a thinning of this structure to minimize the difference to

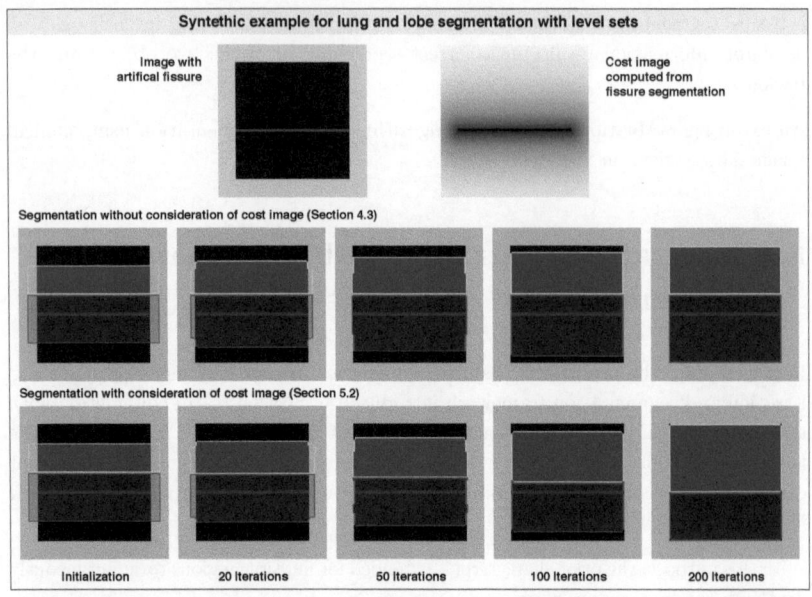

Figure 5.5: Demonstration of lung and lobe segmentation with level sets ($\alpha = 1.0$, $\tau = 0.5$). While lobes are not correctly outlined by the basic level set approach, the inclusion of the cost image using an edge-based term ($\gamma = 10.0$) leads to a correct segmentation.

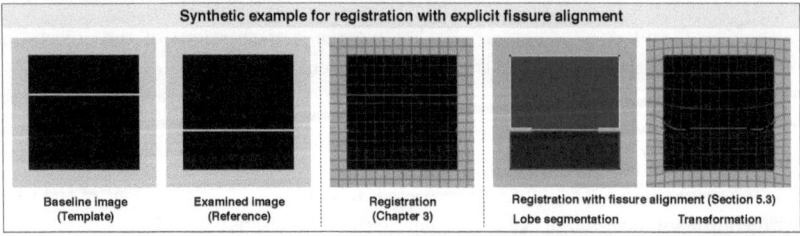

Figure 5.6: With the standard registration approach, a correct alignment of the fissures cannot be achieved, instead only a thinning of the structure can be observed (center image). Integration of a lobe segmentation as described in Section 5.3 results in an almost correct alignment of the fissures. Experiments were performed using semi-implicit diffusion registration with active forces and $\tau_1 = 1.0$, $\alpha_1 = 1.0$, $\beta_1 = 0.25$, $\tau_2 = 0.5$, $\alpha_2 = 0.5$, $\beta_2 = 0.1$, $\gamma = 0.5$ and 500 iterations on three levels.

the reference image (also compare Figure 5.2). Integrating a lobe segmentation approach results in a better alignment of the fissures after registration.

On a side note, an inaccurate motion estimation is observed at the object boundary, which is caused by the homogeneous smoothing. Principally, the inside of the stylized lung moves downwards and the outside remains fixed. In practice, however, the regularizer causes a smooth transition between the motion in both regions. The estimated lung motion is therefore diminished by the non-moving background. As a remedy to this problem, sliding conditions will be introduced in Chapter 6.

The approach for registration with explicit fissure alignment is extensively evaluated in Section 7.4 using clinical image data.

5.4 Discussion

In this chapter, an approach to combine non-linear registration and level set segmentation in a integrated framework was presented. By joining both methods, their mutual dependency is exploited to enhance the results. For example, knowledge about a transformed reference segmentation can be used to avoid leakage of the segmentation into neighboring objects. Vice versa, corresponding segmentations in template and reference image are employed to steer the registration.

Using the joint framework, morphological knowledge can be incorporated in the registration method. This is particularly advantageous in cases where a registration based only on image intensities fails. As demonstrated for lung fissures, shape information provided by a fissure enhancement filter can be considered in the segmentation algorithm and consequently improve registration using the joint framework.

A drawback of the approach is the high number of parameter values that have to be determined. The parameters of the registration (τ_1 and α_1) and segmentation modules (τ_2, α_2 and γ) can be optimized separately according to Chapter 3 and 4. In addition, the parameters β_1 and β_2 are used to determine the influence of segmentation and registration on each other. The optimization of their values is a delicate matter and has to be done application-specifically. It is primarily influenced by the anticipated reliability of the components: For example, if registration accuracy is expected to be good, the influence of the registration on the segmentation can be amplified by choosing a higher value for β_2.

Chapter 6

Sliding motion in image registration

The approach for image registration presented in Chapter 3 aims at finding a transformation that is optimal with respect to a similarity measure and a smoothness condition that ensures a physiologically plausible motion. One of the major challenges for such registration methods in the context of this work is the occurrence of sliding motion – a physiological characteristic that is, for example, observed at the boundaries of multiple structures during the respiratory cycle [Werner et al. 2009a]. In particular, in the case of the breathing-induced lung motion, the outer (parietal) pleura moves in anterior direction following the raise of the ribcage, while the inner (visceral) pleura is pulled in inferior direction by contraction of the diaphragm. The space enclosed between the pleurae – known as the pleural cavity – is filled with a fluid and subject to a pressure below atmospheric pressure, such that both pleurae stay in close contact to each other. When the lung expands, visceral and parietal pleura are therefore sliding along each other (see Figure 6.1) in a (almost) frictionless manner. Recent studies further show that sliding motion not only occurs at the lung boundaries, but also between the individual lung lobes [Sheng and Cai 2008; Ding et al. 2009; Yin et al. 2010; Amelon et al. 2012]. Moreover, organs adjacent to the lung like the liver show the same characteristics [von Siebenthal et al. 2007].

Sliding motion is challenging because it contradicts common regularization models like

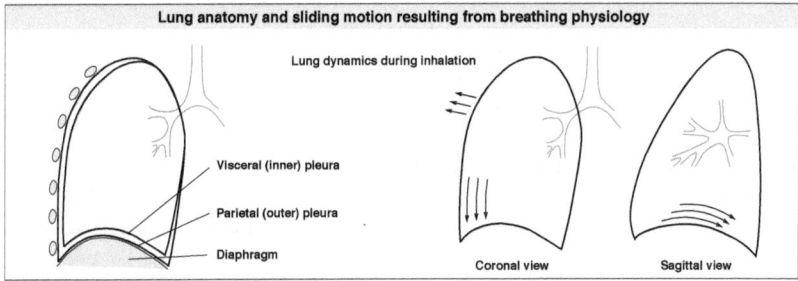

Figure 6.1: Occurance of sliding motion during respiratory lung motion due to a raise of ribcage and a simultaneous contraction of the diaphragm.

diffusion, elastic or Gaussian regularization presented in Section 3.3: While smoothing is required to avoid discontinuities like gaps or foldings in the field, it is defined with the underlying assumption of a globally continuous motion. However, the physiological characteristics of the aforementioned organ imply discontinuities between the motion of organ and surrounding tissue, for example lung and chest wall motion. As a result, registration errors arise in particular near the boundaries of sliding objects.

As mentioned in Chapter 2, the problem of sliding lung motion is usually addressed implicitly by masking the background to prevent it from affecting the force calculation [von Siebenthal et al. 2007; Werner et al. 2009b]. This approach is detailed in Section 6.1. The main contribution of this chapter, however, is the presentation of a novel direction-dependent regularization scheme, which follows in Section 6.2. Utilizing a segmentation, the approach enables a differentiation between different physiological properties: a smooth deformation of the object and sliding motion at its boundaries. Therefore, the model is based on the diffusion regularization as introduced in Section 3.3.1. It is extended to maintain smooth inner-object motion while allowing discontinuities to arise at boundary regions. This is achieved by decoupling normal- and tangential-directed smoothing. Even though developed with an application to lung registration in mind, the presented approach is not limited to this specific field.

After the functionality of masked registration and direction-dependent regularization is demonstrated with some experiments in Section 6.3, the approaches are discussed in the concluding Section 6.4.

6.1 Masked Registration

The most commonly followed approach to reduce errors induced by sliding motion is to restrict registration to the inside of the organs of interest using binary lung masks. This idea is especially appealing for lung registration because very accurate and robust methods exist for the segmentation of this particular organ (see Section 5.2.1). In the inter-institutional study "Evaluation of Methods for Pulmonary Image Registration" (EMPIRE10) conducted by Murphy et al. [2011b], in 16 out of 20 participating methods a masking is applied in at least on step of the algorithm. Among them are the 8 best-rated approaches.

Let $\Sigma_I \subset \Omega$ denote the region of the sliding object in the image I and $S_I : \Omega \to \{0,1\}$ the corresponding segmentation with $S_I(\boldsymbol{x}) = 1$ if $\boldsymbol{x} \in \Sigma_I$ and $S_I(\boldsymbol{x}) = 0$ otherwise. In principle, two closely related approaches for masked registration can be distinguished:

- In several publications, a preprocessing of the images is performed by setting all image values outside the object to a constant $c \in \mathbb{R}$:

$$I^{mask}(\boldsymbol{x}) := I(\boldsymbol{x}) \cdot S_I(\boldsymbol{x}) + c \cdot (1 - S_I(\boldsymbol{x})),$$

with $I \in \{T, R\}$ denoting template and reference image, respectively [Han 2010; Muenzing et al. 2010; Staring et al. 2010; Garcia et al. 2010; Rühaak et al. 2011; Modat et al. 2010a]. The value of c depends on the image content and is chosen for example according to typical background values. This approach requires the segmentations to be very accurate since image information outside the mask is lost. The registration is then performed with R^{mask} and T^{mask} instead of the original images.

- Alternatively, the computation of the update during the registration can be masked by setting the force field outside the object to zero [Schmidt-Richberg et al. 2010a; Song et al. 2010; Cao et al. 2010b]:

$$\boldsymbol{f}^{mask}(\boldsymbol{x}) := \boldsymbol{f}(\boldsymbol{x}) \cdot S(\boldsymbol{x}).$$

In this case, only one segmentation is required that corresponds either to reference or template image, depending on the particular force term: If passive forces with gradients calculated in the reference image are applied, the corresponding mask of the reference image has to be used. Active forces on the other hand utilize gradients of the transformed template image; accordingly, the segmentation of the template image also has to be warped to mask force computation.

In both approaches, registration is limited to the object and provides no information about the transformation of the background. If such information is required as well, the method can be extended by using an inverted mask in a second registration run and combining the resulting deformation fields [Wu et al. 2008; Xie et al. 2009]. Similarly, Yin et al. [2010] assess the slippage between the pulmonary lobes using lobe-by-lobe registration. Besides significantly prolonging computation time, these procedures cannot obviate gaps or foldings along the boundary. While this is partly addressed by Wu et al. [2008] who use a dilated mask, an impact of the background motion to the object motion is reintroduced to a certain degree in this case.

To circumvent the previously mentioned drawbacks, a novel regularization approach is presented in the following to explicitly model the sliding motion along the organ boundaries.

6.2 Direction-Dependent Regularization

Several approaches have been developed that aim at including specific morphological properties in the regularization. Among other works, Loeckx et al. [2004], Pitiot and Guimond [2007], Commowick et al. [2008] and Freiman et al. [2011] apply local rigidity or affine constraints. Kabus et al. [2006] propose to spatially vary regularization parameters to model inhomogeneous elastic properties. Still, none of these approaches addresses the discontinuities arising due to sliding motion.

Nagel and Enkelmann [1986] first presented an anisotropic *image-driven* regularizer for smoothing fields along edges in the image but not across them. This idea was later taken up by Hermosillo et al. [2002]. In medical images, relying only on edges can be insufficient when neighboring objects with similar greyvalues are sliding along each other, for example the liver and its surrounding tissue. Sun et al. [2008] and Zimmer et al. [2009] extended the approach to *joint image- and flow-driven* methods, in which the direction of the regularization is determined by the image while the magnitude depends on the flow. However, these methods origin in computer vision and intend to model the motion of an object in front of the background. Concerning sliding motion in a medical context, the surfaces of object and surrounding tissue remain coherent, that means they cannot overlap and no gaps will arise. This is addressed by a *flow-driven* regularizer proposed by Ruan et al. [2009]. Using a Helmholtz-Hodge decomposition of the displacement field, large shear values are preserved and smaller ones introduced by noise are penalized. While this is a promising approach, a thorough evaluation is lacking. Moreover, all these methods have in common that the resulting smoothness term is applied to the whole image domain, whereas sliding motion only occurs in certain regions. Inside anatomical objects, classical regularization schemes like diffusion or elastic smoothing have been shown to be very suitable [Murphy et al. 2011b].

Also originating in computer vision, a different approach is followed by Brox et al. [2004], who achieve a discontinuity-preserving regularization by penalizing the *Total Variation* (TV) of the flow field, that means the L_1 norm [Rudin et al. 1992]. This approach is extended to a joint registration and motion segmentation framework by Kiriyanthan et al. [2012] and applied to register MR images of the liver.

In this section, a novel *direction-dependent regularization* (DDR) method for modeling sliding organ motion is presented. The approach is formulated as an extension of the diffusion registration, which was introduced in Section 3.3.1 and performs very well for lung registration [Schmidt-Richberg et al. 2010a] (also compare Section 7.2). By decoupling normal- and tangential-directed smoothing, discontinuous sliding motion is allowed to arise at object boundaries while gaps and foldings are prevented. The close connection to diffusion registration allows to restrict sliding motion to these specific regions and to apply the standard regularization elsewhere, such that inner-object motion remains smooth. The method was first introduced in [Schmidt-Richberg et al. 2009b] and is detailed in the following Section 6.2.1. Here, a smooth and accurate segmentation of the organ is needed by the algorithm. To evade this requirement, an extension of the approach is presented in Section 6.2.2: By automatically detecting discontinuities in the motion field, it is possible to spare a prior segmentation and thus do without additional (often manual) expense. Moreover, an extension to multiple

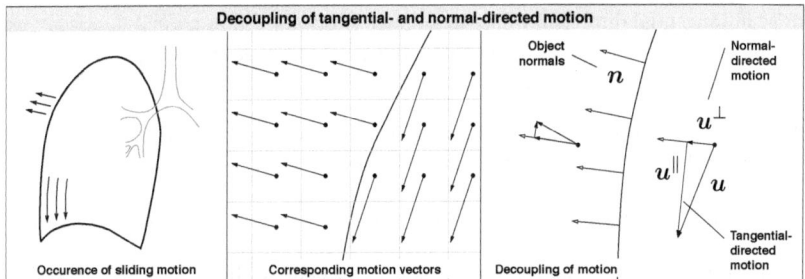

Figure 6.2: In the center image, motion vectors as caused by sliding motion (left) are depicted. These are not smooth in the sense of a globally homogeneous, for example diffusion regularizer. By decoupling $u^\perp$ and $u^\|$ (right), motion at the object boundary can be enforced to be smooth only in normal direction.

objects is presented in Section 6.2.3 to assess – for example – the sliding motion between the pulmonary lobes.

The idea of direction-dependent regularization was recently adopted in other publications, for example by Pace et al. [2011], who formulate the problem as an anisotropic diffusion process or in [Delmon et al. 2011] for a spline-based regularization. Risser et al. [2011] applied a direction-dependent regularization within a piecewise diffeomorphic registration framework.

The section at hand is largely based on the publications [Schmidt-Richberg et al. 2009b, 2010b, 2012a,e].

6.2.1 A direction-dependent regularization model

The diffusion regularization (3.15) is extended by restricting inter-object smoothing to the direction perpendicular to the object Σ that exhibits sliding characteristics. To begin with, a segmentation S_R of the object in the reference image is assumed to be given, which can be obtained using any manual or automatic segmentation algorithm. Specifically for the lung, suitable approaches have been discussed in Section 5.2.1. However, to obtain optimal results, the segmentation has to be as accurate as possible and sufficiently smooth for a robust computation of the object normals. Regardless of the segmentation's origin, a post-processing step according to the level-set-based refinement introduced in Section 4.2.1 is therefore advised. Hereafter, $\phi : \Omega \to \mathbb{R}$ denotes the refined level set function that corresponds to the segmentation S_R.

Knowledge about the motion physiology of organ and surrounding tissue is now incorporated by allowing them to slide along each other. From a technical point of view, discontinuities between the movement of object and background are only allowed to arise in tangential direction, while smoothness is maintained in normal direction (see Figure 6.2). The latter is essential to avoid gaps between or an overlapping of object and background.

To this end, the displacement field $\boldsymbol{u}$ is divided in two components: the normal-directed part $\boldsymbol{u}^\perp$ and the tangential-directed part $\boldsymbol{u}^\|$ with

$$\boldsymbol{u}^\perp(\boldsymbol{x}) = \langle \boldsymbol{u}(\boldsymbol{x}), \boldsymbol{n}(\boldsymbol{x}) \rangle \boldsymbol{n}(\boldsymbol{x}) \qquad \text{and} \qquad \boldsymbol{u}^\|(\boldsymbol{x}) = \boldsymbol{u}(\boldsymbol{x}) - \langle \boldsymbol{u}(\boldsymbol{x}), \boldsymbol{n}(\boldsymbol{x}) \rangle \boldsymbol{n}(\boldsymbol{x}) \,,$$

where $\boldsymbol{n}(\boldsymbol{x})$ denotes the normal on the object at a point $\boldsymbol{x}$. If the level set function of the segmentation is given, the normals can be computed by $\boldsymbol{n}(\boldsymbol{x}) = \nabla \phi(\boldsymbol{x})/\|\nabla \phi(\boldsymbol{x})\|$. The diffusion regularizer (3.15) can then be rewritten as

$$\begin{aligned} \mathcal{S}^{diff}[\varphi] &= \frac{1}{2} \sum_{l=1}^{d} \int_\Omega \|\nabla(u_l^\perp + u_l^\|)\|^2 \, d\boldsymbol{x} \\ &= \frac{1}{2} \sum_{l=1}^{d} \int_\Omega \|\nabla u_l^\perp\|^2 \ + \ \|\nabla u_l^\|\|^2 \, d\boldsymbol{x} \,. \end{aligned} \tag{6.1}$$

As detailed in Appendix B.2, $\boldsymbol{n}$ is assumed to be independent of location in the second step, which allows to write $\sum_{l=1}^{3} \langle \nabla u_l^\perp, \nabla u_l^\| \rangle = 0$. This assumption is feasible because organ surfaces are smooth with respect to image spacing and the gradient of $\boldsymbol{n}$ can therefore be considered to be small.

Based on (6.1), the direction-dependent regularization is defined in two steps. First, the domain of the divided energy term is altered: While a comprehensive (i.e. inter-object) smoothing is to be realized in normal direction, object and background are smoothed separately in tangential direction. Thus, $\|\nabla u_l^\perp\|^2$ is defined as before on the whole image domain Ω but $\|\nabla u_l^\|\|^2$ is restricted to inside and outside the object $\Sigma := \Sigma_R$. This leads to the interim formulation for a direction-dependent regularization

$$\mathcal{S}^{diff}[\varphi] := \frac{1}{2} \sum_{l=1}^{d} \left(\int_\Omega \|\nabla u_l^\perp\|^2 \, d\boldsymbol{x} + \int_\Sigma \|\nabla u_l^\|\|^2 \, d\boldsymbol{x} + \int_{\Omega/\Sigma} \|\nabla u_l^\|\|^2 \, d\boldsymbol{x} \right) .$$

In a second step, a weighting function $\omega : \mathbb{R} \to [0, 1]$ is included to restrict the calculation of the direction-dependent term to the region close to the object borders and to smooth according to the diffusion term (3.15) elsewhere. This is mainly done because normals are only defined along the object boundaries, but it also entails a computational benefit. The final energy term then reads

$$\begin{aligned} \mathcal{S}^{DDR}[\varphi] := \frac{1}{2} \sum_{l=1}^{d} \Bigg(&\int_\Omega \omega \, \|\nabla u_l^\perp\|^2 + (1 - \omega) \, \|\nabla u_l\|^2 \, d\boldsymbol{x} \\ &+ \int_\Sigma \omega \, \|\nabla u_l^\|\|^2 \, d\boldsymbol{x} + \int_{\Omega/\Sigma} \omega \, \|\nabla u_l^\|\|^2 \, d\boldsymbol{x} \Bigg) . \end{aligned} \tag{6.2}$$

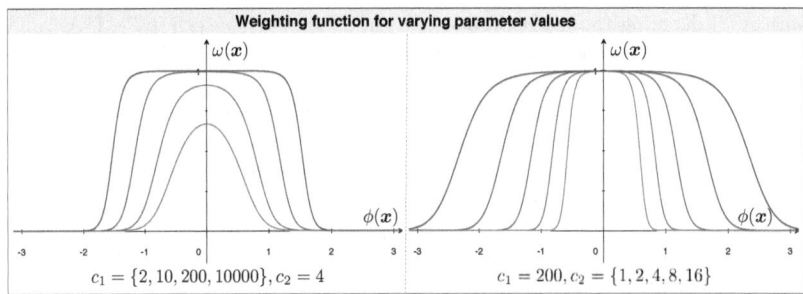

Figure 6.3: Weighting function ω depending on the distance to the zero level set of segmentation ϕ.

Here, the Dirac-shaped weighting function

$$\omega(\boldsymbol{x}) := \delta(\phi(\boldsymbol{x})) := 1 - \frac{1}{1 + c_1 \exp(-c_2\phi(\boldsymbol{x})^2)} \qquad (6.3)$$

proposed by Kabus [2006] is used to determine the object borders, exploiting the fact that $\phi(\boldsymbol{x})$ is defined as the distance of $\boldsymbol{x}$ to the boundary. The constants c_1 and c_2 influence the amplitude and the slope of the function (see Figure 6.3).

In a continuous formulation, the energy (6.2) still equals the diffusion term (3.15). However, differences will arise during the discrete calculation of the derivatives introducing Neumann boundary conditions.

Equivalent to Section 3.1.1, the calculus of variations is utilized to derive the Euler-Lagrange equation of (6.2). As proven in appendix B.1.2.4, this leads to

$$\mathcal{A}^{DDR}[\boldsymbol{u}] = \nabla\omega\nabla\boldsymbol{u}^{\perp} + \nabla(1-\omega)\nabla\boldsymbol{u} + \widehat{\nabla}\omega\widehat{\nabla}\boldsymbol{u}^{\parallel}. \qquad (6.4)$$

Here, $\widehat{\nabla}$ denotes that the gradient is calculated only inside or outside the object, respectively, using Neumann boundary conditions as detailed in the following.

6.2.1.1 Discretization and numerical stability of the DDR scheme

The terms in (6.4) are closely related to the anisotropic diffusion equation $\partial_t\boldsymbol{u} = \nabla\omega\nabla\boldsymbol{u}$ with the diffusivity map ω. To this end, in a first step, the discretization of the corresponding operator $\mathcal{A}^{\omega}$ is derived following Weickert et al. [1998]. In the one-dimensional case and introducing Neumann boundary conditions at the image boundaries, the tridiagonal matrix $A^{\omega} = (a_{ij}^{\omega})$ holds the entries

$$a_{ij}^{\omega} = \begin{cases} \frac{\omega_i+\omega_j}{2h^2} & j \in \mathcal{N}(i), \\ -\sum_{n\in\mathcal{N}(i)} \frac{\omega_n+\omega_i}{2h^2} & j = i, \\ 0 & \text{else} \end{cases} \qquad (6.5)$$

with $\mathcal{N}(i)$ denoting the neighborhood of i. In detail, $\mathcal{N}(i) = \{i+1, i-1\}$ is valid in non-boundary regions and $\mathcal{N}(0) = \{1\}$ for lower and $\mathcal{N}(N) = \{N-1\}$ for upper image boundary, respectively. To obtain a stability threshold for τ, Gershgorin's circle theorem is applied in analogy to Section 3.3.1.1. This leads to $-c_i = r_i = \frac{\omega_{i\pm1} + \omega_i}{2h^2}$ at the boundaries and $-c_i = r_i = \frac{\omega_{i-1} + 2\omega_i + \omega_{i+1}}{2h^2}$ elsewhere. Since $\omega \in [0,1]$, the step size $\tau_{max} = \frac{h^2}{2\alpha}$ is still applicable to maintain numerical stability. The multi-dimensional case can be assembled analogously to Section 3.3.1.1.

In the next step, the direction-dependent regularization (6.4) is examined. The corresponding matrix A^{DDR} can be derived by

$$
\begin{aligned}
A^{DDR}\vec{U} &= A^\omega \vec{U}^\perp + A^{1-\omega}\vec{U} + \hat{A}^\omega \vec{U}^\parallel \\
&= A^\omega N\vec{U} + A^{1-\omega}\vec{U} + \hat{A}^\omega (I - N)\vec{U} \\
&= \left(A^\omega N + A^{1-\omega} + \hat{A}^\omega (I - N) \right) \vec{U}
\end{aligned} \tag{6.6}
$$

with

$$
N := \begin{bmatrix} N_{11} & \cdots & N_{d1} \\ \vdots & \ddots & \vdots \\ N_{1d} & \cdots & N_{dd} \end{bmatrix},
$$

and $N_{kl} \in \mathbb{R}^{N \times N}$ being diagonal matrices holding the product $n_k(\boldsymbol{x}_j) \cdot n_l(\boldsymbol{x}_j)$ in the main diagonal. The matrix $\hat{A}^\omega$ equals A^ω but features Neumann boundary conditions at the object boundaries. In detail, the neighborhood condition in (6.5) is altered to

$$
\widehat{\mathcal{N}}(i) := \{j : j \in \mathcal{N}(i) \wedge S_R(\boldsymbol{x}_i) = S_R(\boldsymbol{x}_j)\}
$$

If $\hat{A}^\omega$ and A^ω were equal (i.e. if there is no sliding object in the image domain), the first and third term in (6.6) would sum up to the anisotropic diffusion matrix A^ω and together with the second term, A^{DDR} would be equal to A^{diff}. Due to the non-trivial structure of the matrix A^{DDR}, an inversion would involve high computation cost. The focus of this work therefore lies on solving the corresponding registration problem with the FED solution scheme. To this end, the maximal time step τ_{max} of the explicit scheme has to be derived in a first step.

After some calculations, it can be shown that in agreement with the previous observations $\lambda_i \in [-\frac{4}{h^2}, 0]$ still holds for rows without voxels corresponding to an object boundary. However, for rows featuring Neumann boundary conditions and again assuming $\nabla \boldsymbol{n}$ to be small, Gerschgorin's circle theorem yields

$$
-c_i = r_i = \frac{2}{h^2} + (1 - n_l^2)(a_{i,i-1}^\omega - a_{i,i+1}^\omega),
$$

with $l \in \{1, \ldots, d\}$. It is known that $(1 - n_l^2) \in [0,1]$ is mostly very small because the normal is orthogonal to the object boundary. While also $(a_{i,i-1}^\omega - a_{i,i+1}^\omega) \in [-1,1]$ is evident, in this case the exact value can be computed depending on the image spacing and the parameters of the function ω. A worst-case estimation leads to a stable step size $\tau_{max} = \frac{h^2}{\alpha(2+h^2)}$.

The final algorithm is summarized in Algorithm 6.1. To guarantee that n is defined and to decrease computation time, A^{DDR} is only calculated for voxels x with $\omega(x) > t_\omega$ for a threshold $t_\omega = 0.001$, and approximated by A^{diff} elsewhere.

Algorithm 6.1 Non-linear registration with direction-dependent regularization.

Set $k = 0$ and $\vec{U}^{(0)}$ to zero.
Compute normal field $\vec{N}$ by $n(x_j) = \nabla\phi(x_j)$ for all j.
Compute weighting function $\omega(x_j)$.
repeat
    Compute passive forces $\vec{F}^{(k)}$.   ▷ Section 3.2
    Let $\vec{U}^{(k)} \leftarrow \vec{U}^{(k)} - \tau\vec{F}^{(k)}$.
    Compute $\vec{U}^{\perp(k)}$ and $\vec{U}^{\parallel(k)}$.
    Let $\vec{U}^{(k)} \leftarrow \vec{U}^{(k)} + \tau\alpha\left(A^\omega\vec{U}^{\perp(k)} + A^{1-\omega}\vec{U}^{(k)} + \widehat{A}^\omega\vec{U}^{\parallel(k)}\right)$.
    Let $k \leftarrow k + 1$.
until algorithm converges or $k = k_{max}$.

6.2.2 DDR with automatic detection of discontinuous motion

To avoid the requirement for a known segmentation, an alternative approach for automatic detection of slipping organ motion is presented in this section. To do so, knowledge about the motion physiology is incorporated by making certain assumptions. In detail, it is assumed that

a) sliding organ motion occurs only along edges in the image,

b) image gradients are approximately orthogonal to the organ surface, and

c) sliding motion is directed alongside an edge in the image.

These assumptions are thoroughly discussed in Section 6.4. The approach consists of three steps. First, candidate voxels – that means voxels at which sliding motion may potentially occur – are automatically detected in the image, followed by an image-based computation of object normals. Then, the amount of sliding motion is quantified by sampling displacement vectors close to candidate voxels. These steps are detailed in the following.

To apply a scheme like (6.4), Neumann boundary conditions have to be used at object borders. With respect to assumption a), a Deriche edge detection algorithm is used to find boundaries in the image [Deriche 1987]. In this method, an edge is defined as pixels with gradient magnitudes above a certain threshold. Moreover, the edge is restricted to the local maximum of that value in gradient direction to suppress non-maximum responses, which is crucial to restrain edges to one pixel in width. Since edges found by this algorithm are not always closed, the image domain cannot be divided into disjunct regions in a straightforward manner. Instead, boundary conditions are applied between edge voxels $\mathcal{C}^{edge}(\Omega)$ and voxels $\mathcal{C}^{adj}(\Omega)$ that are adjacent to edge voxels in the direction of the image gradient. Together, they define the set of candidate voxels $\mathcal{C}(\Omega)$ at which sliding motion can potentially occur.

In a second step, object normals are computed. According to assumption b), these are equal to the normalized gradient of the reference image

$$n(x) := \frac{\nabla \left(R * G_\sigma(x) \right)}{\left\| \nabla \left(R * G_\sigma(x) \right) \right\|} \, .$$

To improve robustness, the image is smoothed before normal computation by convolution with a Gaussian filter kernel G_σ with standard derivation σ. This does not influence the edge localization, which is done beforehand.

The weighting function is determined in a third step. Instead of defining ω depending on the distance to the object boundary as done in (6.2.1), the weight is used to quantify to what extent motion exhibits sliding characteristics. It is the intention to use direction-dependent regularization only in regions with discontinuous motion like the outer lung pleurae, while a diffusion regularization is applied near the hilum. This is done to increase robustness, since sliding motion does not occur at every edge in the image. Let

$$u_n(x) := \frac{u(x + rn(x)) \; - \; u(x - rn(x))}{2r}$$

with a radius r be the motion variation in normal direction, which is an approximation of the directional derivative of u in direction n. According to assumption c), sliding motion implies that u_n lies in the plane orthogonal to n. Therefore, for $\|u_n\| \neq 0$ the amount of sliding motion is quantified depending on the angle θ between u_n and n, with

$$\cos(\theta) := \frac{\langle n, u_n \rangle}{\|u_n\|} \, .$$

The weighting function ω is then defined as

$$\omega(x) := \begin{cases} \left(1 - \cos(\theta)^{2c_1}\right)^{c_2} & \text{if } x \in \mathcal{C}(\Omega) \text{ and } \|u_n\| \neq 0 \\ 0 & \text{else} \end{cases} \, . \tag{6.7}$$

The constants c_1 and c_2 determine the slope of the curve and therefore the tolerance against angle differences. Their influence is depicted in Figure 6.4.

The estimation of the normal-directed variation of motion u_n is challenging because discontinuities arise at object boundaries. Therefore, a sampling of motion vectors is proposed as illustrated in Figure 6.4. Let $x_j^\pm := [x_j \pm rn(x_j)]$ be neighbors of a voxel $x_j \in \mathcal{C}(\Omega)$ in positive and negative normal direction within a certain distance r, where $[\cdot]$ denotes a rounding to the closest grid point. Normal-directed motion variation is

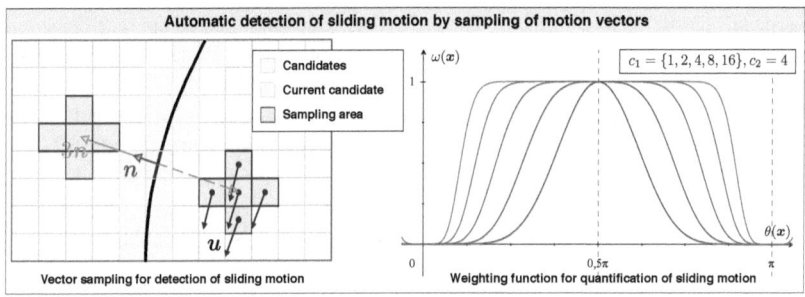

Figure 6.4: After candidate voxels for sliding motion are detected (grey voxels), mean motion is sampled in positive ($u^+(x_j)$) and negative ($u^-(x_j)$) normal direction (blue regions). The amount of sliding motion is quantified using the weighting function on the right depending on the angle θ between u_n and n. Illustration following [Schmidt-Richberg et al. 2012e].

then estimated by $u_n := (u^+ - u^-)/2r$ with

$$u^\pm(x_j) := u * K(x_j^\pm),$$

where K is an arbitrary smoothing kernel, for example $K := G_\sigma$. The convolution is used instead of simply regarding $u(x_j^\pm)$ to get a less locally confined estimation of the motion and therefore increase the robustness of the algorithm. Experiments suggest that a mean filtering in a 6-neighborhood provides a reasonable trade-off between computational efficiency and accuracy. To avoid interpolation across edges, the radius r is then chosen such that x_j is not part of the regions around x_j^+ and x_j^- used for sampling (here $r = 3$).

6.2.3 DDR with multiple objects for modeling lobe sliding

As previously mentioned, sliding motion is also observed between the pulmonary lobes (see Chapter 5 for an explanation of lobe anatomy); Ding et al. [2009] even report sliding distances of up to 20 mm. By meshing each lobe individually and adding sliding conditions between them, Sheng and Cai [2008] were able to significantly improve a biophysical model for respiratory motion estimation. Ding et al. [2009] and Amelon et al. [2012] applied a lobe-by-lobe registration to assess lobe sliding. With the same aim, a spatially varying regularization weight was used by [Yin et al. 2010], leading to an anisotropic-diffusion-like approach.

In this section, the use of direction-dependent regularization for modeling sliding lobe motion is examined. An automatic detection of discontinuous motion as presented in Section 6.2.2 is not applicable in this context because the underlying assumptions are violated: Neither are edges visible between the lobes, nor are image gradients necessarily perpendicular to the lobe surfaces. Therefore, the segmentation-based approach (Section 6.2.1) has to be extended to be able to handel multiple objects. To this end, in analogy to Section 4.3 the object Σ is split in $N-1$ disjunct sub-objects Σ_i, $i = 1, \ldots, N-1$, with $\bigcap_i \Sigma_i = \emptyset$ and $\bigcup_i \overline{\Sigma_i} = \overline{\Sigma}$. Further, $\Sigma_0 := \Omega \setminus \overline{\Sigma}$ denotes the background region. Using this notation, the energy term for a direction-dependent regularization (6.2) can be reformulated to

$$\mathcal{S}^{DDR}[\varphi] := \frac{1}{2} \sum_{l=1}^{d} \left(\int_{\Omega} \omega \, \|\nabla u_l^{\perp}\|^2 + (1 - \omega) \, \|\nabla u_l\|^2 \, d\boldsymbol{x} + \sum_{i=0}^{N-1} \int_{\Sigma_i} \omega \, \|\nabla u_l^{\parallel}\|^2 \, d\boldsymbol{x} \right).$$

(6.8)

Here, the weighting function ω and the normals $\boldsymbol{n}$ at a point $\boldsymbol{x}$ are computed using the level set function ϕ_i of the corresponding region Σ_i by

$$\boldsymbol{n}(\boldsymbol{x}) := \sum_{i=0}^{N-1} \left(1 - H(\phi_i(\boldsymbol{x})) \right) \frac{\nabla \phi_i(\boldsymbol{x})}{\|\nabla \phi_i(\boldsymbol{x})\|}$$

and

$$\omega(\boldsymbol{x}) := \sum_{i=0}^{N-1} \left(1 - H(\phi_i(\boldsymbol{x})) \right) \delta(\phi_i(\boldsymbol{x})),$$

where H denotes the Heaviside function as introduced in Chapter 4. Given this, the algorithm detailed in Algorithm 6.1 is used.

6.3 Experiments

To illustrate the impact of sliding motion on image registration, synthetic images as shown in Figure 6.5 are examined. The first example exhibits a sliding in horizontal direction. In the second example, inside and outside of a circle are rotated by 10 degree in opposing directions. In each experiment, the standard diffusion registration is compared to a masked registration (Section 6.1) and the proposed direction-dependent regularization.

In both examples, diffusion regularization entails a cross-boundary smoothing of the transformation, which contradicts motion physiology and leads to errors in this region. This effect is reduced using a masked registration. However, the resulting transformation is valid only inside the object. Moreover, the untransformed outer part slows convergence and a considerably higher number of iterations is required to reach a correct transformation. The direction-depend approach yields correct displacements in the whole image domain. However, minor interpolation errors can be observed in the second example, which will be discussed in the next section.

In a second experiment illustrated in Figure 6.6, direction-dependent regularization with automatic detection of sliding motion as presented in Section 6.2.2 is applied. Since the

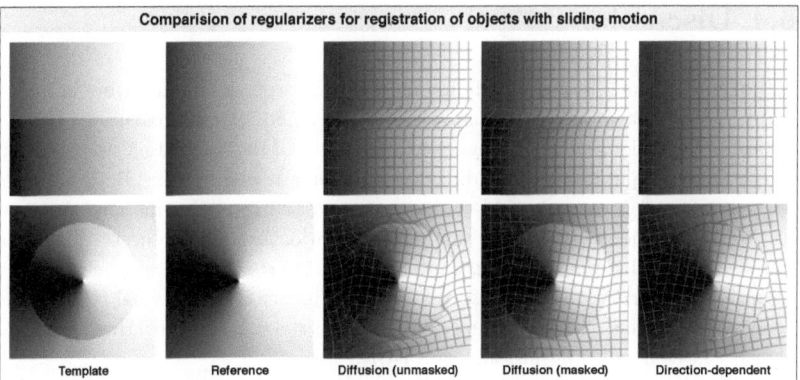

Figure 6.5: Comparison of direction-dependent regularization with masked and unmasked diffusion regularization (upper half and inner circle are defined as object for the masked registration). All experiments are performed with active forces, $\alpha = 0.5$ $\tau = 0.125$ and $k_{max} = 1000$ iterations. The explicit solution scheme is applied.

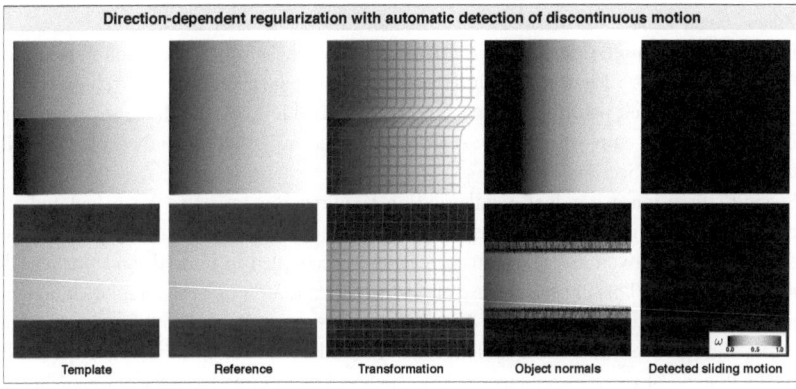

Figure 6.6: Direction-dependent regularization with automatic detection of sliding motion. All parameters were chosen as in Figure 6.5 and additionally $\sigma = 2.0$ for the computation of object normals.

underlying assumptions are violated (no edges at object boundary, no image gradients perpendicular to surface), detection fails in the first example. As a consequence, diffusion regularization is applied on the whole image domain. In the second example, however, sliding motion is detected as intended and the correct transformation is computed.

6.4 Discussion

As pointed out in this chapter, sliding motion can cause significant errors in image registration if not properly accounted for. To this end, two approaches have been presented to consider breathing physiology: a masking of the registration (in particular, of the force computation) and a direction-depending regularization. Both methods have the potential to considerably reduce errors caused by sliding motion. However, masked registration only yields a valid transformation inside the object. While this can be obviated by repeating registration with an inverted mask and combining the resulting transformations, such process implies a higher computational effort. This problem aggravates with the number of objects in the image. In contrast, multiple objects can be handled intrinsically with DDR.

While both masked registration and direction-dependent regularization generally require a segmentation of the sliding object, an extension has been presented for the latter approach to evade this requirement by automatically detecting the occurrence of sliding motion in the transformation. However, this pragmatic approach relies on underlying assumptions and fails if these are not met. The applicability in practice therefore has to be demonstrated using clinical data, which is done extensively in Section 7.5.

From an algorithmic point of view, two major drawbacks of the direction-dependent regularization exist. First, due to the complex structure of the matrix A^{DDR}, application of the semi-implicit solution scheme (3.8) is not possible in a straightforward manner. For clinical data, employment of Fast Explicit Diffusion is therefore advisable and will be considered in Section 7.5.

Second, direction-dependent regularization requires the forces to be calculated in the domain of the reference image R, that means in the same image in which the segmentation is given and the transformation is decoupled in normal- and tangential-directed motion. This implies the use of passive forces that "pull" the template image to fit the reference image (see Section 3.2). However, as shown in Section 3.5, using passive forces can go along with some undesired effects and active or "pushing" forces defined in the domain of the target image perform slightly better in practice [Schmidt-Richberg et al. 2009a].

As shown in the second example in Figure 6.5, artifacts can arise at surfaces with high curvature. The reasons for this are twofold: On the one hand, the assumption that n is independent of x is violated in such regions, which can potentially affect the computed transformation. On the other hand, interpolation errors may arise since displacement vectors close to convex surfaces can point to the other region without violating the smoothness condition.

Chapter 7

Evaluation with clinical image data

In theory, there is no difference between theory and practice.
But, in practice, there is.

Jan L. A. van de Snepscheut

To assess the applicability of the presented algorithms in a clinical setting, the focus of this chapter lies on an in-depth evaluation based on actual CT data.

After a specification of the materials and methods used throughout this chapter, the basic registration framework is evaluated for the alignment of thoracic CT images in Section 7.2. In detail, considered fields of application cover motion estimation using 4D image data (Section 7.2.2), inter-subject registration for atlas generation (Section 7.2.4) and intra-patient registration (Section 7.2.3), whereof the latter is based on the results of the international evaluation study EMPIRE10. These studies aim at comparing the accuracy of the registration algorithm on the level of its components. In this way, appropriate modules can be chosen for different scenarios in the subsequent evaluations. In Section 7.3, the approach for pulmonary lobe segmentation presented in Section 5.3 is analyzed, and in the following Section 7.4 its integration in the joint registration and segmentation framework. Finally, the focus of Section 7.5 lies on the evaluation of direction-dependent regularization for modeling sliding motion (see Chapter 6).

7.1 Materials and methods

To establish a basis for the subsequent evaluation studies, the utilized materials and methods are detailed in tis section. First, after a brief introduction to CT imaging, the image data used throughout this chapter is characterized. Subsequently, metrics for a quantitative evaluation are explained.

7.1.1 Practical aspects of CT imaging

Electromagnetic radiation in the form of x-rays has first been systematically studied by Wilhelm Röntgen in 1895. Enabling the visualization of the inside of the human body, x-rays quickly started to occupy an increasingly important role in medical imaging. However, since traditional radiograms are projection images and therefore object to superimposition, they only provide limited information about the spatial distribution of objects. This problem was resolved with the invention of *Computed Tomography* (CT) in the early 1970s, which made the acquisition of axial slice images possible. Here, a series of data scans is progressively taken from different angles by rotating the x-ray source – usually together with the opposing detector – around the object. Based on this data, slice images free of superimposition are computed using a reconstruction algorithm like the dual Radon transformation, linear algebra techniques or an iterative approach based on expectation-maximization.

The evaluation studies presented in this chapter are entirely based on clinical CT images. The focus of this section therefore lies on the specification of some properties of this imaging modality that are of relevance for the following examinations. A profound introduction to CT imaging can be found for example in [Buzug 2008; Kalender 2011].

Image values and Hounsfield Units   The image value associated to each voxel is a measure of the material's radiodensity, that means the inability of electromagnetic radiation to pass through the particular tissue. For example, structures like bones absorb most of the x-rays, such that only little radiation is measured at the detector. Soft tissue, in contrast, is less attenuating. Voxel values are standardized according to the Hounsfield scale. *Hounsfield Units* (HU) of water and air are defined to be 0 HU and -1000 HU, respectively, that means 1 HU represents a change of 0.1% of the attenuation coefficient of water. Other clinically relevant values are around -900 HU to -500 HU for the lung and +20 HU to +50 HU for the heart, and +60 HU to +70 HU for the liver [Buzug 2008].

Due to this specification, CT scans acquired with different imaging devices are comparable to each other. This entails that – besides calibration errors between different devices and anatomical deviations – the greyvalue probability distributions of a specific object required for the region-based segmentation approach are transferable from one device to the other and from one patient to the other.

Reconstruction of volumetric images   Early CT scanners acquired images a single slice at a time. After a full gentry rotation, the motorized table on which the patient lies was moved in axial direction and the next slice was assessed. Advances in technology allowed the installation of more than one detector array in the scanner, enabling the acquisition of multiple slices with one rotation. The physical distance between the detector rings determines the slice thickness of the image. Single slices or segments of multiple slices – current scanners typically vary between 4 and 64 slices – are then composed to obtain a volumetric image. However, if the object is deformed during acquisition of neighboring segments (in particular due to breathing motion), image quality is impaired by step artifacts. This problem is slightly moderated by spiral CT scanners operating in *helical mode*, in which the x-ray tube continuously rotates around the patient.

Reconstruction of 4D images For the 4D CT images regarded in this work, each image segment was acquired multiple times per table position, aiming for full coverage of the breathing cycle. Additionally, scans were correlated with a breathing signal obtained using, for example, an abdominal belt or a spirometer. In this way, each segment can be assigned to the corresponding point in the breathing cycle.

Volumetric images are reconstructed for a particular time point or lung volume by assembling appropriate segments for each table position. Most commonly this is done using the nearest-neighbor principle, that means the segment with the volume closest to the desired volume is regarded for reconstruction. This procedure usually introduces severe reconstruction artifacts between the segments when the actual volume differs considerably from the intended volume. To this end, a more sophisticated approach was presented by Ehrhardt et al. [2007], in which segments are interpolated for the specific volume using an optical-flow-based approach.

Radiation dose and image quality To acquire CT images, the definition of technical parameters of the scanner like beam energy, tube current, exposure time or table speed (in helical mode) is necessary, which is always a tradeoff between high image quality and low radiation exposure [McNitt-Gray 2004]. Radiologists therefore have to aim at minimizing the applied dose while ensuring an image quality sufficiently high for the clinical purpose at hand (for example, the detection of lung emphysema requires a higher quality than the localization of lung tumors).

A way to reduce the applied dose is for example to decrease the tube current or exposure time (measured in mAs, milliampere times exposure time), which directly reduces the number of emitted x-ray photons. However, image noise – measured as standard deviation of voxel values in a homogeneous material like water – is proportionally increased by this procedure. Varying the voltage of the x-ray tube (kVp, kilovolt peak) also influences the dose but entails differences in image contrast and susceptibility to image artifacts. Other factors like the table pitch or axial increment also influence the dose but are restricted by the intended slice thickness after reconstruction.

The problem of dose reduction is aggravated for the acquisition of 4D images because multiple scans are acquired per couch position. For example, while 400-700 mAs are common for normal-dose 3D scans, Low et al. [2003] use only 40 mAs for each scan acquired to reconstruct a 4D sequence to reduce the total radiation dose.

7.1.2 Considered image data

For the subsequent studies, different pools of proprietary as well as publicly available CT images have been considered. These are detailed in the following. Furthermore, available supplemental data like landmarks or segmentations required for quantitative evaluation is listed (see Section 7.1.3). An illustrative overview on the images including specifications about size, resolution and the scanner parameters is given in Figure 7.1.

WashU The WashU image pool contains twelve proprietary 4D CT data sets of lung tumor patients and was established in cooperation with the Washington University School of Medicine in St. Louis, MO, USA. The images were acquired with a step-and-shoot protocol during free breathing and reconstructed using the optical flow based method at 10 to 14 time points during the respiration cycle [Ehrhardt et al. 2007]. Details on the imaging protocol are given in [Low et al. 2003].

For all images, lung segmentations were generated using a basic region-growing approach with subsequent manual correction. Moreover, on average 80 corresponding landmarks were determined by a clinical expert in maximum inhalation and maximum exhalation, aiming for equal distribution in the lung.

DIR-Lab This set of ten publicly accessible 4D CT images is hosted by DIR-lab, University of Texas M. D. Anderson Cancer Center, TX, USA, with the aim of providing *"the medical imaging community with a comprehensive repository of reference standard data sets for objective and rigorous evaluation of deformable image registration spatial accuracy performance"* [Castillo et al. 2009]. The data sets are available under `http://www.dir-lab.com/`. They were recorded from patients treated for esophageal cancer with a step-and-shoot cine protocol and reconstructed retrospectively using the nearest neighbor principle. While all images were acquired with the same scanner, half of them (cases 01 to 05) were cropped at the rib cage and subsampled in-plane to 256×256 pixels.

For each image, lung segmentations were generated using an automatic intensity-based approach [Wilms et al. 2012]. Additionally, a set of 300 landmarks per image is provided by the hosts. These landmarks were selected by an expert in medical imaging, visually reviewed a second time and their location adjusted if necessary. In the process, uniform spatial distribution of the landmarks was ensured.

POPI The "Point-validated Pixel-based Breathing Thorax Model" (POPI) is hosted by the Léon Bérard Cancer Center & CREATIS lab, Lyon, France [Vandemeulebroucke et al. 2007] and available under `http://www.creatis.insa-lyon.fr/rio/popi-model/`. The data set was acquired using a 16 slice CT and sorted using the nearest neighbor principle. A belt strapped around the thorax was used as external signal for synchronization.

Lung segmentations were generated using an automatic intensity-based approach [Wilms et al. 2012]. A set of 41 manually selected landmarks is provided by the hosts for each image. However, most of the landmarks are placed close to the bronchial tree and some even outside the lung. Therefore, a supplemental set is examined, in which outer-lung landmarks were excluded and additional landmarks manually selected, aiming for equal distribution (landmarks per image).

EMPIRE10   The EMPIRE10 ("Evaluation of Methods for Pulmonary Image Registration 2010") challenge is an ongoing contest with the aim of comparing different algorithms for the registration of lung CT images. The intention of the challenge is to provide a *"public platform for fair and meaningful comparison of registration algorithms, which are applied to a database of intra-patient thoracic CT image pairs"* [Murphy et al. 2011b]. The EMPIRE10 study is discussed in more detail in Section 7.2.3.

The data pool considered in the challenge is publicly available and consists of 30 image pairs, on which the results in Section 7.2.3 are based. The scans originate from several different sources and include 8 breath-hold inspiration scan pairs, 8 breath-hold inspiration and expiration scan pairs, 4 4D data scan pairs (only end inhalation and end exhalation are considered), 4 ovine data scan pairs, 2 contrast to non-contrast scan pairs, and 4 artificially warped scan pairs. All pairs have been cropped to contain just the lung region. For more details of the applied imaging protocols including dose, image size, and resolution, the reader is referred to the challenge website `http://empire10.isi.uu.nl/` or the respective publication.

Lung segmentations are provided for each image. However, landmarks and lobe segmentations of the 30 data sets are not publicly available since evaluation and comparison is performed by the organizers of the challenge.

RUKSH   This set of nine thoracic normal-dose 3D CT images was acquired at the Clinic for Radiology and Nuclear Medicine, University Hospital Schleswig-Holstein, Lübeck, Germany. The normal dose data sets (120 kVp, 450-750 mAs) with a high resolution of $0.79 \times 0.79 \times 0.7$ mm exhibit a relatively high visibility of the lung fissures and are therefore used to evaluate the lobe segmentation algorithm presented in Section 5.2. The images were cropped to the lung region to reduce computation time.

The lungs were automatically segmented using the same intensity-based approach as before [Wilms et al. 2012]. Lobe segmentations were generated as ground truth for evaluation using a spline-based interpolation of manually determined fissure points inspired by Wang et al. [2006] and a subsequent manual correction.

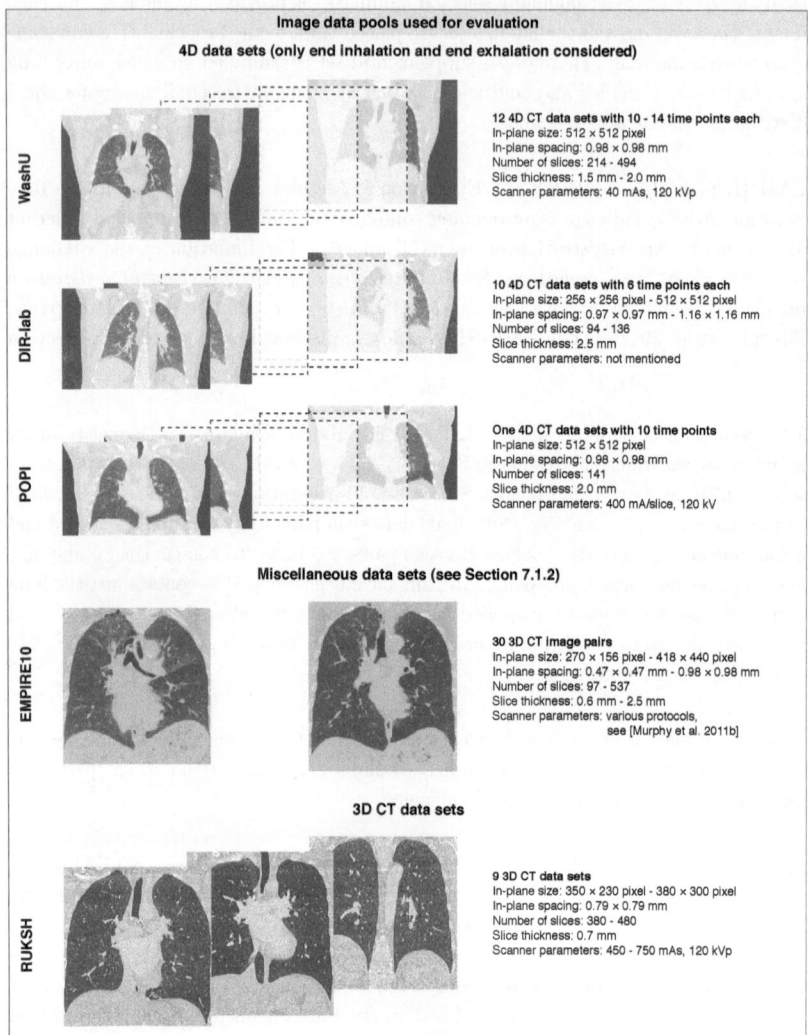

Figure 7.1: Overview on the image data considered for the evaluation studies presented in this chapter, including specifications of image size, resolution and the applied tube current and energy. The DIR-lab, POPI and EMPIRE10 data sets are publicly available and therefore suited as a standard evaluation platform.

7.1.3 Metrics for evaluation of segmentation and registration results

To allow an objective evaluation and comparison of registration and segmentation results, several metrics are introduced that can be used to quantify their accuracy.

7.1.3.1 Metrics for quantifying segmentation accuracy

In the following, let $S : \Omega \rightarrow \{0,1\}$ denote the result of an automatic segmentation algorithm and $M : \Omega \rightarrow \{0,1\}$ a manually generated reference segmentation (also called ground truth). Let further $\mathrm{Seg}(\Omega)$ be the set of all possible segmentations over Ω. A metric

$$\mathcal{M}^{Seg} : \mathrm{Seg}(\Omega) \times \mathrm{Seg}(\Omega) \rightarrow \mathbb{R}$$

is then defined to quantify the similarity between two segmentations.

Overlap coefficients Most commonly used for quantifying segmentation similarity are overlap coefficients like the Jaccard (or Tanimoto) index and the closely related Dice coefficient

$$\mathcal{M}^{Dice}[S, M] := \frac{2 \cdot |\{\boldsymbol{x}_j \in \Omega^{\#} : S(\boldsymbol{x}_j) = M(\boldsymbol{x}_j) = 1)\}|}{|\{\boldsymbol{x}_j \in \Omega^{\#} : S(\boldsymbol{x}_j) = 1\}| + |\{\boldsymbol{x}_j \in \Omega^{\#} : M(\boldsymbol{x}_j) = 1\}|} , \tag{7.1}$$

which is considered in this work. Here, $\Omega^{\#}$ denotes the set of discrete grid points (see Appendix A). However, thoughtfulness is required for interpreting overlap coefficients because they only depend on the number of misclassified voxels and not their remoteness from the reference segmentation. Moreover, large and compact objects exhibit larger overlap coefficients because the fraction of overlapping volume is generally higher than for small objects.

Mean and maximal surface distance To counter the restrictions of the overlap coefficients, the mean and maximal surface distance between automatic and manual segmentation is often regarded. Let $\mathcal{B}(S)$ be the set of boundary pixels of S with

$$\mathcal{B}[S] := \{\boldsymbol{x}_j \in \Omega^{\#} : S(\boldsymbol{x}_j) = 1 \wedge (\exists\, i \in \mathcal{N}(j) : S(\boldsymbol{x}_i) = 0)\}$$

and $\mathcal{N}(j)$ being the set of indices neighboring to index j. The mean and maximal surface distance are then defined as

$$\mathcal{M}^{Mean}[S, M] := \frac{1}{|\mathcal{B}[S]|} \sum_{\boldsymbol{x}_j \in \mathcal{B}[S]} \mathrm{dist}(\boldsymbol{x}_j, \mathcal{B}[M]) , \tag{7.2}$$

and

$$\mathcal{M}^{Max}[S, M] := \max_{\boldsymbol{x}_j \in \mathcal{B}[S]} \mathrm{dist}(\boldsymbol{x}_j, \mathcal{B}[M]) , \tag{7.3}$$

respectively, where dist($\boldsymbol{x}_j, \mathcal{B}[M]$) is the Euclidean distance of voxel $\boldsymbol{x}_j$ to the closest voxel of $\mathcal{B}[M]$. The metric was symmetrized by interchanging S and M in a second run and regarding the average.

Lobe and fissure distances If an image contains multiple objects – for example the five pulmonary lobes, see Chapter 5 – the aforementioned metrics can be applied to each object individually. For the specific case of lobe segmentation, however, additional and physiologically more meaningful metrics are commonly regarded [van Rikxoort et al. 2010].

Let $\boldsymbol{S} = (S_i)_{i=1,\ldots,N}$ be the vector containing the segmentations S_i of each of the N objects. With $\mathcal{B}_{k,l}[\boldsymbol{S}]$ the set of voxels of object S_k that lie at the boundary to object S_l is described:

$$\mathcal{B}_{k,l}[\boldsymbol{S}] := \left\{ \boldsymbol{x}_j \in \Omega^\# : S_k(\boldsymbol{x}_j) = 1 \land (\exists\, i \in \mathcal{N}(j) : S_l(\boldsymbol{x}_i) = 1) \right\}.$$

Using this set, the mean fissure distance (and equivalently the maximal distance) can be defined as above by

$$\mathcal{M}_{k,l}^{Mean}[\boldsymbol{S}, \boldsymbol{M}] := \frac{1}{|\mathcal{B}_{k,l}[\boldsymbol{S}]|} \sum_{\boldsymbol{x}_j \in \mathcal{B}_{k,l}[\boldsymbol{S}]} \text{dist}(\boldsymbol{x}_j, \mathcal{B}_{k,l}[\boldsymbol{M}]). \tag{7.4}$$

Moreover, an additional metric is introduced in the style of [Murphy et al. 2011b]. It aims at quantifying the proportion of the lobe boundaries that are successfully traced in the segmentation result:

$$\mathcal{M}_{k,l}^{Fiss}[\boldsymbol{S}, \boldsymbol{M}] := \frac{|\{\boldsymbol{x}_j \in \Omega^\# : \boldsymbol{x}_j \in \mathcal{B}_{k,l}[\boldsymbol{M}] \land \boldsymbol{x}_j \in \mathcal{B}_{k,l}^+[\boldsymbol{S}]\}|}{|\{\boldsymbol{x}_j \in \Omega^\# : \boldsymbol{x}_j \in \mathcal{B}_{k,l}[\boldsymbol{M}]\}|}. \tag{7.5}$$

Here, to incorporate some tolerance, the fissure region $\mathcal{B}_{k,l}$ is expanded by ± 3 voxels in cranio-caudal (CC) direction and denoted by $\mathcal{B}_{k,l}^+$.

7.1.3.2 Metrics for quantifying registration accuracy

Quantifying registration accuracy is challenging because the true transformation is generally not known on the whole image domain. Therefore, to rate registration results, different strategies are pursued in current literature [Sarrut et al. 2007; Castillo et al. 2009; Murphy et al. 2011b]: In monomodal image registration, basic intensity-based metrics are considered to rate the similarity between reference and transformed template image. Moreover, the accuracy of the transformation is estimated by the degree of alignment of certain structures – defined by segmentations or landmarks – after registration. Finally, properties of the transformation itself, like invertibility and inverse consistency, are regarded as measurements of the plausibility of the transformation.

Intensity-based metrics   The most straightforward approach to evaluate the accuracy of monomodal CT registration is to assess the intensity differences between reference and transformed template image. For example, the *Root of Mean Squares* (RMS) is defined by

$$\mathcal{M}^{RMS}[R,T;\varphi] := \left(\frac{1}{N} \sum_{j=1}^{N} \left(R(\boldsymbol{x}_j) - T \circ \varphi(\boldsymbol{x}_j) \right)^2 \right)^{\frac{1}{2}}. \tag{7.6}$$

Alternative formulations are the *Sum of Squared Differences* (SSD) or the *Mean Squared Difference* (MSD), which are not further regarded as metrics in this work.

Segmentation metrics for registration   If two segmentations S_R and S_T of an object in reference and template image are known, the metrics introduced in Section 7.1.3.1 can be used to implicitly assess registration quality by measuring the similarity between reference and transformed template segmentation:

$$\mathcal{M}^{Reg}[S_T, S_R; \varphi] := \mathcal{M}^{Seg}[S_T \circ \varphi, S_R].$$

Landmark Alignment Error   Further, the alignment of corresponding characteristic points – so-called landmarks – is evaluated after registration. Such landmarks depict for example bifurcations of blood vessels and are usually manually determined by a medical expert in reference and template image. To obtain a meaningful and unbiased estimation of registration accuracy, landmarks have to be available in a sufficient number and as equally distributed over the image domain as possible [Castillo et al. 2009; Kabus et al. 2009].

Let $\boldsymbol{l}_R = (\boldsymbol{l}_{R,l})_{l=1...,L}$ be an array containing the coordinates $\boldsymbol{l}_{R,l} \in \Omega$ of L landmarks in the reference image and let $\boldsymbol{l}_T$ be the corresponding landmark positions in the template image. The mean *Landmark Alignment Error*[1] (LAE) is then defined as

$$\mathcal{M}^{LAE}[\boldsymbol{l}_R, \boldsymbol{l}_T; \varphi] := \frac{1}{L} \sum_{l=1}^{L} \|\boldsymbol{l}_{T,l} - \varphi(\boldsymbol{l}_{R,l})\|. \tag{7.7}$$

Landmark-based evaluation is very common for intra-patient registration and can be regarded as the *status quo* methodology. However, in the inter-patient case it is often not applicable because annotating a sufficient number of anatomically corresponding points is impracticable.

Jacobian determinant   The determinant of the Jacobi matrix of the transformation –

---

[1] The Landmark Alignment Error is also called *Target Registration Error* (TRE) in many publications. However, this notation is avoided here to prevent confusion with the term that describes the misalignment of a target structure after point-based rigid-body registration of fiducials [Fitzpatrick and West 2001].

also called Jacobian determinant or simply Jacobian – is given by

$$\det(\nabla\varphi(\boldsymbol{x})) = \left| \begin{bmatrix} \frac{\partial\varphi_1(\boldsymbol{x})}{\partial x_1} & \frac{\partial\varphi_1(\boldsymbol{x})}{\partial x_2} & \frac{\partial\varphi_1(\boldsymbol{x})}{\partial x_3} \\ \frac{\partial\varphi_2(\boldsymbol{x})}{\partial x_1} & \frac{\partial\varphi_2(\boldsymbol{x})}{\partial x_2} & \frac{\partial\varphi_2(\boldsymbol{x})}{\partial x_3} \\ \frac{\partial\varphi_3(\boldsymbol{x})}{\partial x_1} & \frac{\partial\varphi_3(\boldsymbol{x})}{\partial x_2} & \frac{\partial\varphi_3(\boldsymbol{x})}{\partial x_3} \end{bmatrix} \right|$$

in the three-dimensional case. It is used to assess the change of volume in an infinitesimal neighborhood of a point $\boldsymbol{x}$: A value $\det(\nabla\varphi(\boldsymbol{x})) > 1$ implies an expansion of volume, $0 < \det(\nabla\varphi(\boldsymbol{x})) < 1$ indicates a contraction [Rey et al. 2002]. If $\det(\nabla\varphi(\boldsymbol{x})) = 0$, all points in the neighborhood of $\boldsymbol{x}$ are mapped to a single point, which implies a singularity in the transformation. For $\det(\nabla\varphi(\boldsymbol{x})) < 0$, the orientation of the local coordinate system at point $\boldsymbol{x}$ is changed and a folding occurs. Therefore, the Jabcobian determinant is used to define a measure for the plausibility of the transformation by calculating the number of voxels with a negative value or a value of zero:

$$\mathcal{M}^{Jac}[\varphi] := \left| \{\boldsymbol{x}_j \in \Omega^{\#} : \det(\nabla\varphi(\boldsymbol{x}_j)) \le 0\} \right|. \tag{7.8}$$

In practice, it is often more convenient to assess the Jacobian of the displacement field instead of the transformation. Since $\varphi(\boldsymbol{x}) = \boldsymbol{x} - \boldsymbol{u}(\boldsymbol{x})$, the condition can then be reformulated to $\det(\nabla\boldsymbol{u}(\boldsymbol{x})) \ge 1$.

Inverse Consistency Error   The symmetry error or *Inverse Consistency Error* (ICE) can be assessed by performing a second registration run with interchanged template and reference image [Christensen and Johnson 2001]. Ideally, the transformations yielded by forward and backward registration should be inverse to each other. However, in practice differences occur, which are regarded as an indicator for implausible results. The inverse consistency error is therefore defined by

$$\mathcal{M}^{ICE}[\varphi_{R\to T}, \varphi_{T\to R}] := \frac{1}{N} \sum_{j=1}^{N} \|\varphi_{T\to R}(\varphi_{R\to T}(\boldsymbol{x}_j)) - \boldsymbol{x}_j\|, \tag{7.9}$$

where $\varphi_{R\to T}$ is the result of the registration with R as reference image and $\varphi_{T\to R}$ the computed transformation with interchanged template and reference image.

7.1.3.3 Assessing statistical significance

To further characterize the difference between two algorithms, a two-sample t-test can be performed considering the metric values $\mathcal{M}$ for each patient of a data pool. A statistically significant improvement is constituted at a value of $p \le 0.05$.

It should be noted that in case of the landmark alignment error, different strategies exist in the literature for performing the t-test. Sarrut et al. [2007] propose to test the individual landmark distances for each patient independently. However, this approach provides a statement about significance for each data set and not the collective. Therefore, Castillo et al. [2009] apply the test on the total of landmarks of all images but this approach is biased if the number of landmarks varies between the patients. In this work, tests on statistical significance are therefore performed – in accordance with the other metrics – considering the mean landmark alignment errors $\mathcal{M}^{LAE}$ of each patient.

7.2 Problem-specific composition of algorithms for lung registration

In this section, the registration framework presented in Chapter 3 is evaluated for lung CT registration with different areas of application.

To begin with, some application-specific details of the algorithm that apply to all studies are clarified in Section 7.2.1. The core evaluation is then divided in three parts.

First, intra-patient registration with the aim of motion estimation is regarded in Section 7.2.2. Here, template and reference image are different time points of a 4D data set and the computed transformation represents the motion of tissue during the depicted physiological process, which – in case of lung CT images – is the respiratory motion.

The general case of intra-patient registration is analyzed in Section 7.2.3 with regard to the results of the EMPIRE10 challenge. While the considered images still originate from the same subject, they were acquired at different sessions and/or with different imaging devices, for example during a follow-up study to monitor the progression of a disease. The primary goal is therefore not the estimation of the patient's motion but the alignment of different scans.

In the third case, inter-patient registration is analyzed, which aims at establishing correspondences between the anatomy of different subjects (see Section 7.2.4). This task mainly emerges for atlas-based segmentation techniques.

7.2.1 Implementation details

In the following, some sophistications of the algorithm are presented that are applied to obtain best registration accuracy and performance.

7.2.1.1 Histogram matching

The distance measures presented in Section 3.2 are based on the assumption of constant greyvalues. This assumption might be violated in practice due to greyvalue derivations caused by tissue compression, the use of different scanners or – in case of inter-patient

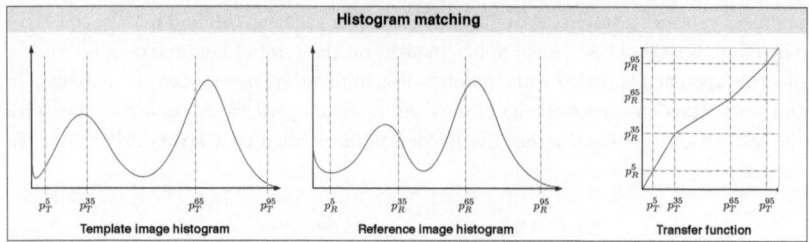

Figure 7.2: Illustration of a histogram matching with $B = 4$ bins. First, the quantiles p_I^5, p_I^{35}, p_I^{65} and p_I^{95} are computed in for template (left) and reference image (center). The transfer function m (right) is a piecewise linear function that maps the quantiles of the template to the reference image.

registration – anatomical anomalies. Therefore, a histogram matching is performed to achieve maximal registration accuracy.

The algorithm for histogram matching applied in this work is inspired by [Nyúl et al. 2000]. Let $h_I : \mathbb{R} \to \mathbb{R}$ be the histogram of image I with

$$h_I(g) := |\{\boldsymbol{x}_j \in \Omega^\# : -0.5 < I(\boldsymbol{x}_j) - g \le 0.5\}|.$$

Furthermore, let p_I^P with $0 \le P \le 100$ denote the P-th percentile of histogram h_I, that means the smallest value, below which P percent of the greyvalues in the image are found. To match the histograms h_R and h_T of reference and template image, first a number of B bins is determined in the histograms as the percentiles

$$p_I^{5+90\cdot b/(B-1)}, \qquad b = 0, \dots, B-1\,.$$

The percentiles p_I^5 and p_I^{95} are used as limits instead of the maximal and minimal greyvalue to avoid a bias caused by outliers, for example metal artifacts. In the next step, a piecewise linear matching function $m : \mathbb{R} \to \mathbb{R}$ is defined that matches the bins of T to the bins of R such that $h_R \approx h_{m(T)}$. Registration is then performed with R as reference and $m(T)$ instead of T as template image. The process of histogram matching is illustrated in Figure 7.2.

7.2.1.2 Stop criterion

A second aspect with a huge impact in practice is the choice of the stop criterion, which is used to constitute convergence in the Algorithms 3.1, 3.5, 5.1, and 6.1. In general, the state of convergence is reached if a defined metric $\mathcal{M}^{Stop}$ that measures the accuracy of the transformation implies no further improvement of the registration.

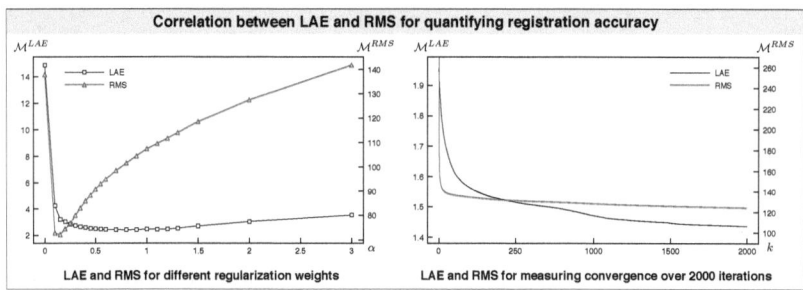

Figure 7.3: Left: Low correlation between LAE and RMS for different regularization weights: While RMS indicates an optimal α of about 0.2, LAE is lowest for $\alpha = 0.8$. Right: Low correlation between LAE and RMS for constituting convergence: LAE convergences after considerably more iterations than RMS.

Several choices exist for the definition of $\mathcal{M}^{Stop}$. Theoretically, the most adequate measure would be the energy functional (3.2), that means $\mathcal{M}^{Stop} := \mathcal{J}^{Reg}$. However, the energy can be computationally expensive to evaluate and is therefore not always considered in practice.

As a simplification, the Root of Mean Squares $\mathcal{M}^{RMS}$ can be regarded, which can be assessed at minimal cost during the computation of the force term $\boldsymbol{f}$. This approach is followed in this work. Peroni et al. [2011] discuss several alternative choices but none proved to be significantly superior.

While principally all metrics introduced in Section 7.1.3.2 can be incorporated in the stop criterion as well, the landmark alignment error is recognized to be most reliable for quantifying registration accuracy. This is addressed in [Schmidt-Richberg et al. 2011], where $\mathcal{M}^{LAE}$ is used as metric for the stop criterion employing a set of automatically detected landmarks. The idea is based on the observation, that LAE and RMS are not well correlated as shown in Figure 7.3 (left). This leads to the effect that while the RMS has already reached a state of convergence during the iterative registration process, the LAE continues to decrease and thus indicates further improvement of the registration result (see Figure 7.3, right). Accordingly, the landmark alignment error can indeed provide more reliable information about the state of convergence than the MSD. However, landmarks for the computation of $\mathcal{M}^{LAE}$ are not always at hand and an automatic detection might not be possible for all types of image data. Therefore, this approach is not further followed in this work but it could potentially lead to improved registration results.

In this work, the registration algorithm is stopped if no improvement of $\mathcal{M}^{Stop}$ is achieved in the course of k^{Stop} iterations (here: $k^{Stop} = 10$). On the finest level, however, this approach can be very time consuming due to the high computational cost of each iteration and the slow convergence of the registration. Therefore, on this level a least squares linear regression on the MSD values of the 20 most recent iterations is

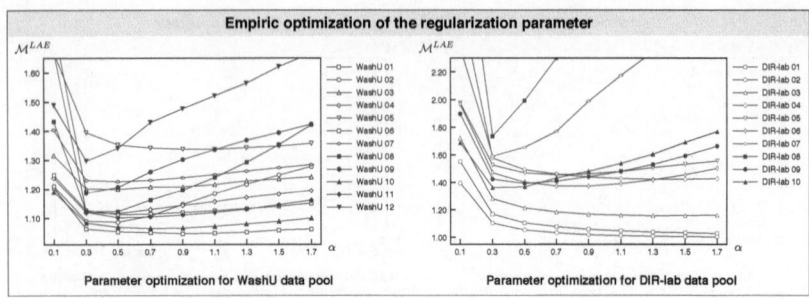

Figure 7.4: For each individual scan pair, the LAE is given for the registration with different values of α. While the registration of the WashU images exhibits a relatively constant response to the value alpha, the optimal value for the DIR-lab pool strongly varies.

performed. If the slope of the fitted line is below a certain threshold (here: $t^{Slope} = 10^{-4}$), registration is aborted.

In case FED is utilized, meaningful metric values can only be assessed at the end of complete cycles. This is considered in the stop criterion by adapting k^{Stop} and t^{Slope} in proportion to the number of iterations per cycle, such that it is as comparable as possible to the stopping conditions for the other schemes.

7.2.1.3 Parameter optimization for registration

In the basic registration framework, the values of only two substantial parameters have to be determined, the step size τ and the regularization weight α.

For the explicit solution scheme, τ is principally given by the theoretical stability limit. However, in practice slightly larger values are still stable and provide better results, which can be explained by a reduced risk of getting stuck in a local minimum. Therefore, an empiric optimization is performed using training data, aiming for the smallest landmark alignment error without an increased value of $\mathcal{M}^{Jac}$. The same strategy is followed for the step size in the semi-implicit scheme.

The parameter α is likewise optimized. As the experiments in Figure 7.4 demonstrate, the optimal value for this weight can considerably vary from case to case. Therefore, the value with the smallest mean $\mathcal{M}^{LAE}$ is chosen to register all images.

An alternative is presented in [Schmidt-Richberg et al. 2011]. Again utilizing automatically detected landmarks, $\mathcal{M}^{LAE}$ is evaluated to adapt the weight during the registration process. Using such an automatic case-specific optimization, considerably better registration results can be achieved, especially for heterogeneous image pools like the DIR-lab data. However, apart from the high computational cost, the restrictions for employing automatically detected landmarks highlighted in the preceding section also apply. Therefore, this approach is not further pursued in this work.

7.2.2 Intra-patient registration of 4D images for motion estimation

As initially discussed, motion estimation is one of the major fields of application for non-linear registration. From a methodical point of view, registering time points of 4D data sets can be regarded as the most elementary task because it entails several advantages: First, images are well aligned, such that no pre-registration of the image domains is required. Second, the imaging device used for data acquisition is identical for all time points, that means no calibration errors arise and tissue compression is the only cause of greyvalue deviations between reference and template image. Moreover, anatomy is only influenced by physiological motion and not by the usual daily variations of organ shape and volume caused by, for example, a different intestinal content.

7.2.2.1 Study setup

Based on these observations, the first and most elementary study aims at evaluating and comparing the individual components of the registration framework presented in Chapter 3 with application to motion estimation. These modules are in detail:

1. **Distance Measure:** SSD vs. active NSSD forces vs. passive NSSD forces vs. dual NSSD forces.

2. **Regularization:** Diffusion vs. Elastic.

3. **Transformation space:** Standard vs. diffeomorphic vs. symmetric diffeomorphic framework.

4. **Physiological properties:** Masked vs. unmasked registration.

5. **Solution scheme:** explicit vs. semi-implicit vs. FED.

The comparison of points 1.-4. is thoroughly performed in [Werner 2012]. That study is based on the WashU, DIR-lab and POPI data sets. From every data set, maximal inhalation and maximal exhalation were chosen as reference and template image, respectively, and registration was performed for each of the 48 possible combinations of the modules (4 force terms, 2 regularizers, 3 transformation spaces, masked/unmasked). For all registration runs, the semi-implicit solution scheme was chosen with the parameters $\tau = 1.0$, $\alpha = 0.5$ (NSSD), $\tau = 2.5 \cdot 10^{-6}$, $\alpha = 0.1$ (SSD), $\lambda = \mu = 0.5$ for elastic regularization and $k_{max} = 800$ (NSSD) or $k_{max} = 2400$ (SSD).

To avoid redundancy, the study conducted by Werner [2012] is not repeated at this point. Instead, only the key findings are summarized. The focus of this section is on point 5., the comparison of the solution schemes. Based on the best-performing algorithm identified by Werner [2012], registration was performed with explicit, semi-implicit and FED schemes on the image pools WashU, DIR-lab and POPI. Parameter values of step size and regularization weight have been optimized empirically for the explicit scheme ($\tau = 0.2$, $\alpha = 0.07$). Even though this step size is slightly larger than τ_{max} and therefore bears the risk of numerical instability, it provides the best results in practice and is therefore considered for comparison. For FED, τ_i were computed based on τ_{max} as derived in Section 3.3.1.2 with a cycle time $T = 5.0$. All results were compared with regard to registration accuracy $\mathcal{M}^{LAE}$, plausibility $\mathcal{M}^{Jac}$ and processing time.

7.2.2.2 Results

The key findings of the study described by Werner [2012] can be summarized as follows:

- **Force computation:** Masked registration significantly outperforms unmasked forces in all cases. On average, the LAE is reduced by 0.8 mm ($p \leq 0.001$). This effect is explained by an under-estimation of the lung motion due to the sliding characteristics at the boundary – see Chapter 6 and Section 7.5 for more details. Moreover, the normalization in the formulation of NSSD forces entails a better alignment of inner-lung structures, which results in a significantly lower LAE then with SSD forces (on average 1.3 mm, $p \leq 0.001$). The differences between the three NSSD formulations is relatively small with a slight but non-significant superiority of active forces (see Figure 7.5). However, the Inverse Consistency Error $\mathcal{M}^{ICE}$ is smallest for $\boldsymbol{f}^{dual}$ with 0.6 mm before $\boldsymbol{f}^{act}$, $\boldsymbol{f}^{pass}$ (both 0.8 mm) and $\boldsymbol{f}^{SSD}$ (1.0 mm).

- **Regularizer:** The difference between elastic and diffusion regularization are principally small, as illustrated in Figure 7.6. Quantitatively, the LAE is about 0.1 mm smaller for $\mathcal{D}^{Diff}$ than for $\mathcal{D}^{Elas}$. This distinction is mainly caused by a slightly worse performance of the elastic regularization in combination with SSD forces – for NSSD forces, the differences are even smaller. A minor superiority of the elastic term is examined with regard to $\mathcal{M}^{Jac}$.

- **Transformation space:** As expected, visual assessment shows that the smoothness of the computed transformation increases from the non-diffeomorphic to the diffeomorphic framework and further to the symmetric diffeomorphic approach (see Figure 7.7). This is confirmed by the evaluation of the Jacobian determinant: $\mathcal{M}^{Jac}$ is zero for all diffeomorphic registration results.
  The increased smoothness entails a slightly reduced accuracy, which manifests in

Table 7.1: Results for the registration with explicit, semi-implicit and FED solution scheme. The mean $\mathcal{M}^{LAE}$ and the standard deviation per data pool are given. The second part of the table shows the results of a second experiment, in which the registration is stopped prematurely after 10 (DIR-lab, POPI) or 15 (WashU) minutes. All registrations are performed with masked NSSD forces, diffusion regularization and the non-diffeomorphic framework. In contrast to [Werner 2012], a value of $t^{slope} = 10^{-4}$ is employed to increase computation speed. Results are detailed for the DIR-lab data in Appendix C.

Dataset	No Reg.	Explicit	FED	Semi-implicit
	– Registration until convergence –			
WashU	6.59 ± 1.78	1.34 ± 0.23	1.36 ± 0.21	$\mathbf{1.30 \pm 0.18}$
DIR-lab	8.46 ± 3.33	1.83 ± 0.58	1.58 ± 0.37	$\mathbf{1.53 \pm 0.29}$
POPI	7.15	1.06	1.05	$\mathbf{1.04}$
	– Registration for 15 (WashU) / 10 (DIR-lab, POPI) minutes –			
WashU	6.59 ± 1.78	1.61 ± 0.35	$\mathbf{1.47 \pm 0.27}$	1.55 ± 0.31
DIR-lab	8.46 ± 3.33	2.14 ± 0.87	$\mathbf{1.77 \pm 0.58}$	1.90 ± 0.68
POPI	7.15	1.10	$\mathbf{1.05}$	1.07

a by 0.1 mm better value of $\mathcal{M}^{LAE}$ (for non-diffeomorphic/diffeomorphic as well as diffeomorphic/symmetric diffeomorphic registrations).

In summary, no universally superior approach can be identified and the best-suited method rather depends on the specific requirements of the application. Elastic regularization slightly outperforms diffusion regularization with respect to accuracy but has a higher computational cost. Diffeomorphic approaches entail a minor loss of accuracy but are beneficial if the inverse transformation is required. A clear recommendation can only be given for the normalization in the formulation of NSSD forces, which significantly outperform SSD-based forces. Moreover, the use of lung masks is obligatory to achieve best accuracy. Based on these observations, quantitative results for the best combination are given as $\mathcal{M}^{LAE} = 1.16$ mm (WashU), 1.34 mm (DIR-lab) and 0.99 mm (POPI).

The studies carried out in the context of this work focus on the remaining comparison between the different solution schemes. The quantitative results of the evaluation are given in Table 7.1. Deviations from the results given in [Werner 2012] solely stem from a more strictly defined stop criterion ($t^{slope} = 10^{-4}$ instead of 10^{-5}) to reduce computation time.

Confirming the observations made in Section 3.5.3, the semi-implicit scheme outperforms the explicit scheme and FED. The improvement is statistically significant with a significance level of $p \leq 0.01$. FED yields considerably but not significantly better results than the explicit scheme.

Registration with the semi-implicit scheme takes on average 10.5 minutes on an Intel Xeon machine with 2.67 GHz. Contrary to the expectations, registration with FED

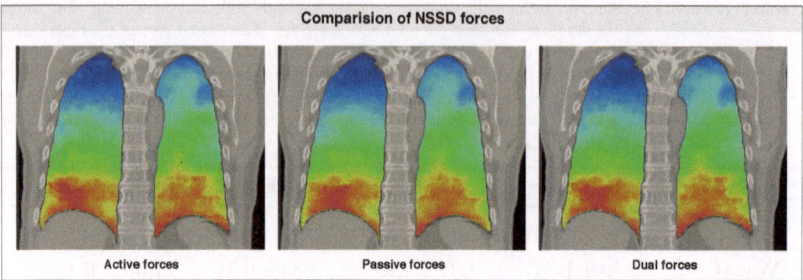

Figure 7.5: Comparison of the motion fields obtained with different formulation of NSSD forces. The color indicates the motion amplitude. Left: active forces (3.12) using gradients of the transformed template image. Center: Passive forces (3.13) using gradients of the reference image. Right: Dual forces (3.14), which are a combination of active and passive forces. Visual differences between the formulations are small.

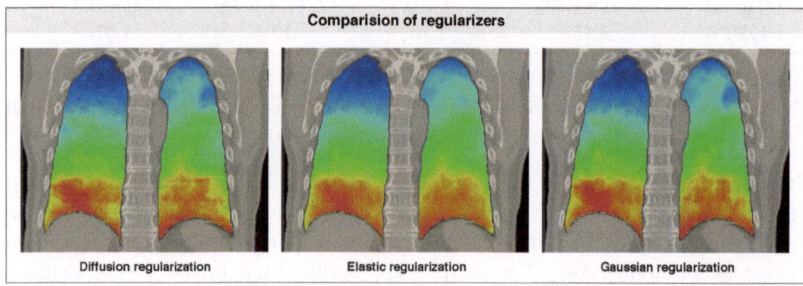

Figure 7.6: Comparison of different regularization approaches. Left: Diffusion regularization (3.15). Center: Elastic regularization (3.21). Right: Gaussian smoothing as described in Section 3.3.3. Only minor differences are visible, for example a smoother appearance of the elastic approach.

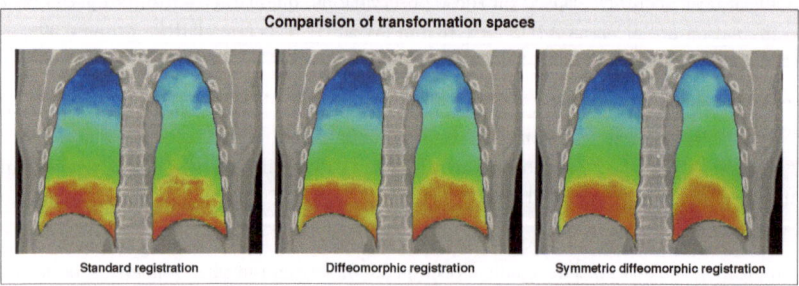

Figure 7.7: Comparison of different transformation spaces. Left: standard registration framework (3.2). Center: Diffeomorphic framework after Section 3.4. Right: Diffeomorphic framework with symmetric forces (3.23). The degree of smoothness is visibly increased from left to right.

(on average 11 minutes) takes slightly longer than with the explicit scheme (9 minutes). This is due to the automatic stop criterion: Using the explicit scheme, registration stops after considerably less iterations than with FED because $\mathcal{M}^{RMS}$ no longer decreases – presumably because registration gets stuck in a local minimum. Using FED, however, minima can be bypassed by iterations with large step sizes.

To avoid this bias and to demonstrate the faster convergence of the FED scheme, a second registration run is performed, in which the computation is stopped after a maximal run time (complete FED cycles are maintained). Thus, a similar number of iterations is performed with the explicit as with the FED scheme, but considerably less with the semi-implicit scheme, which requires more time per iteration. Computation time was set to 10 (DIR-Lab, POPI) and 15 (WashU) minutes, whereat different values are chosen to cope with the varying image sizes. In this experiment, FED performs best of all approaches because it converges faster than the explicit scheme and requires less time per iteration than the semi-implicit scheme. However, the improvement is not statistically significant.

In summary, a semi-implicit scheme should be employed in case computation time is not crucial. If time matters or if the semi-implicit scheme is not applicable for complex regularization approaches (see Chapter 6), FED is superior to the explicit scheme.

7.2.3 Intra-patient registration: The EMPIRE10 study

After evaluating the individual modules of the registration framework, the next step is a comparison with other potentially completely different registration approaches. To this end, an algorithm was composed based on the results of the preceding section and submitted to participate at the EMPIRE10 challenge.

The EMPIRE10 ("Evaluation of Methods for Pulmonary Image Registration 2010") challenge originally took place in the course of the MICCAI 2010 conference in Beijing, China, but is intended to be an ongoing contest. The motivation of the challenge is to provide a standardized evaluation platform for registration results: By testing various algorithms on the same set of data and analyzing the results with the same criterions, an objective comparison between the methods is enabled.

A detailed overview on the challenge results is given in [Murphy et al. 2011b].

7.2.3.1 Study setup

The EMPIRE10 challenge consisted of two phases. The first phase – referred to as offline phase – started in early 2012 when the first 20 data sets were provided by the organizers. Participants had the opportunity to perform the registrations in their own facilities and submit the computed displacement fields to the organizers for evaluation. Phase two – the online phase – took place in the course of the MICCAI workshop[2], Beijing, China, 2010, where the participants registered the remaining 10 data sets within a given time frame of three hours.

For evaluation, four aspects were considered by the organizers:

- **Alignment of Lung Boundaries:** Lung segmentations were generated using the approach of van Rikxoort et al. [2009] and manually corrected, if necessary. Alignment error was quantified as the number of voxels with a distance to the surface of above 2 mm tolerance. The mediastinal region was excluded from the observation.

- **Alignment of Major Fissures:** Pulmonary fissures were extracted using the approach proposed by van Rikxoort et al. [2008]. Their alignment is quantified by a metric very similar to (7.5), but excluding the minor fissure of the left lung and the region with a maximal distance of 20 mm to the lung boundary.

- **Correspondence of Annotated Landmark Pairs:** A set of 100 equally-distributed landmarks was defined in each image using an semi-automatic approach [Murphy et al. 2011a]. Mean landmark distance is defined as in (7.7).

- **Singularities in the Displacement Field:** Discontinuities were detected in the displacement field by assessing the Jacobian determinant according to (7.8).

All submitted results were ranked per image and per metric. The average rank was then considered for the final ranking of the participating algorithms.

7.2.3.2 Details of the algorithm

With the aim of participation at the EMPIRE10 challenge, a registration algorithm consisting of three steps was composed. The algorithm is detailed in [Schmidt-Richberg et al. 2010a].

Pre-registration Since numerous image pairs in the EMPIRE collective were acquired with different scanners or in different sessions (see Section 7.1.2), their coordinate systems potentially deviate considerably from each other. Therefore, a pre-registration consisting of an affine alignment and a non-linear surface registration was employed, which is detailed in [Ehrhardt et al. 2010].

Both steps were based on the binary lung masks $S_T, S_R : \Omega \to \{0, 1\}$ of template and reference image. While these were provided for the EMPIRE10 study, they could also be generated using any of the automatic approaches described in Section 5.2.1. Surface

---

[2] http://www.grand-challenge.org/index.php/MICCAI_2010_Workshop, verified Nov. 2012.

models of the lungs were constructed from the lung segmentation masks using the *Marching Cubes* algorithm [Lorensen and Cline 1987] followed by a triangle decimation and a surface smoothing to obtain surfaces with smooth normals and to reduce the computational complexity of subsequent steps.

In a first step, the surface models of template and reference image were coarsely aligned in an affine pre-registration step using the *Iterative-Closest-Point* (ICP) algorithm [Besl and McKay 1992]. Secondly, the resulting affine transformation φ^{aff} was used as initialization for a symmetric non-linear surface registration algorithm related to the *Geometry-Constrained Diffusion* presented in [Andresen and Nielsen 2001]. The resulting point correspondences were then used to generate a dense transformation φ^{pre} based on a *Thin Plate Spline* (TPS) interpolation.

Stop criteria of the individual steps were chosen as follows: The affine ICP registration stops either after a maximal number of iterations ($k_{max} = 50$) or if the mean vertex distance is below a threshold ($t = 0.01\,\text{mm}$). The same holds for the non-linear surface registration, where $k_{max} = 50$ and $t = 10^{-5}\,\text{mm}$ were chosen.

Diffeomorphic non-linear registration For the core registration step, the presented registration framework was used to compose an algorithm with regard to the findings described in Section 7.2.2 and taking the evaluation metrics of the challenge into account:

- The **non-symmetric diffeomorphic framework** was chosen because discontinuities were to be avoided but inverse consistency was not demanded.

- **Masked active NSSD forces** were favored due to their superiority with regard to registration accuracy.

- To improve processing time, **diffusion regularization** was given preference over the elastic approach.

- The **semi-implicit scheme** was applied to solve the registration problem.

Initialization On the whole, the algorithm can be seen as the concatenation of three registration steps: an affine alignment, a surface-based adjustment and the image-based diffeomorphic registration. In principle, each step can be initialized with the results of the preceding one. However, the further velocity vectors of the diffeomorphic non-linear registration point outside the domain Ω of the fixed image, the more notable extrapolation errors occur during calculation of the exponential map $\exp(\boldsymbol{v})$. This is especially considerable for the scaling-and-squaring algorithm, but also holds for other implementations, e.g. the Euler step approach [Bossa et al. 2008].

As a result, the diffeomorphic registration was not initialized with the result of the pre-registration φ^{pre}. Instead, the reference image R was registered with the warped image

$T^{pre} := T \circ \varphi^{pre}$. By this, velocities and accordingly the extrapolation error remains comparatively small. To calculate the final displacement field, the resulting transformation φ^{diff} was concatenated with φ^{pre} using linear interpolation.

7.2.3.3 Results

In a field of 34 participants, the presented algorithm achieved a fourth place in the offline phase of the challenge, that means for the registration of the first 20 data sets [Schmidt-Richberg et al. 2010a]. The official results are listed in Table 7.2. Equally a fourth place was reached in the online phase for the registration of the remaining 10 data sets, which summed up to a third place overall. The results are detailed in [Murphy et al. 2011b].

On average, the best accuracy was reached with respect to landmark and fissure alignment. In the category of lung boundary alignment, in particular approaches that explicitly accounted for this matter were slightly superior. Moreover, in three of the test cases singularities occurred in the displacement fields, which were introduced by the point-based surface registration and the TPS interpolation. This entailed a comparably bad placement in this category.

7.2.4 Inter-patient registration for atlas generation

In this section, the registration of images from different subjects is analyzed, which can be seen as the most challenging task due to the potentially large anatomical differences between the patients. Inter-subject registration has two major fields of application, atlas generation and (multi-) atlas segmentation.

As motivated in Chapter 1, atlas generation is a common task in computational anatomy. It is aimed at transforming multiple patients to a common reference frame in order to establish correspondences between the subjects. This enables the computation of statistics on the patients' anatomies, for example to assess the mean shape or intensity of an object or intensity variations of a voxel [Younes et al. 2009; Ehrhardt et al. 2011].

In atlas-based segmentation, multiple segmented patient data sets are registered to an image of interest. A segmentation of this image is then composed of the transformed atlas segmentations using a specific atlas selection strategy. This is usually done with respect to the similarity between regarded image and transformed atlas or the amount of deformation between both images [Aljabar et al. 2009].

The intention of this section is to investigate the principle applicability of the presented registration framework in the context of atlas generation and/or atlas-based segmentation. The section is, however, not aimed at presenting a new atlas generation

Table 7.2: Challenge outcome (phase 1) for the submitted algorithm as provided by the organizers. The table shows the results for each scan pair, per category and overall. Rankings and final placement are from a total of 34 competing algorithms.

Scan Pair	Lung Boundaries Score	Rank	Fissures Score	Rank	Landmarks Score	Rank	Singularities Score	Rank
01	0.00	7.00	0.00	2.00	2.12	9.00	0.00	24.00
02	0.00	11.00	0.00	15.00	0.35	4.00	0.00	12.50
03	0.00	5.50	0.00	12.50	0.33	5.00	0.00	12.00
04	0.00	7.00	0.00	16.50	0.97	10.00	0.00	14.00
05	0.00	13.00	0.00	16.00	0.00	5.50	0.00	13.50
06	0.00	16.00	0.00	21.00	0.38	17.00	0.00	14.00
07	0.04	18.00	0.32	4.00	1.46	5.00	0.00	10.00
08	0.00	10.00	0.00	7.00	0.75	7.00	0.00	12.50
09	0.00	5.00	0.00	6.50	0.53	5.00	0.00	13.00
10	0.00	6.00	0.00	15.00	1.20	9.00	0.00	13.50
11	0.00	11.00	0.00	8.00	0.66	6.00	0.00	11.50
12	0.00	28.00	0.00	13.50	0.00	5.00	0.00	14.50
13	0.00	10.00	0.06	4.00	0.86	10.00	0.00	26.00
14	0.01	10.00	2.01	5.00	1.79	6.00	0.00	9.50
15	0.00	8.00	0.00	7.00	0.65	14.00	0.00	12.50
16	0.00	8.00	0.04	12.00	0.97	8.00	0.00	13.50
17	0.00	6.50	0.04	7.50	0.67	4.00	0.00	14.00
18	0.07	20.00	0.07	3.00	2.25	10.00	0.00	10.50
19	0.00	14.00	0.00	12.00	0.61	21.00	0.00	14.50
20	0.11	23.00	1.97	9.00	1.26	4.00	0.00	21.00
Avg	0.01	11.85	0.22	9.82	0.89	8.22	0.00	14.32
Average Ranking Overall								11.05
Final Placement								4

technique – other more sophisticated methods exist and are likely to be better suited in a clinical scenario [Wolz et al. 2010]. Instead, as a proof-of-concept study, the registration algorithm is employed in a basic scheme for atlas generation. The generated atlas is also used in Section 7.3 for a coarse initialization for the presented lobe segmentation approach. A similar algorithm is further employed in [Ehrhardt et al. 2011] for the generation of a mean motion model.

7.2.4.1 Study setup

Two studies were conducted, both based on the RUKSH data set featuring 9 normal-dose CT scans of different patients (see Section 7.1.2).

Pairwise registration In the first study, pairwise registration of all images was performed, resulting in 72 registrations in total. The specific registration approach equals the method used in the EMPIRE10 study (masked active NSSD forces, diffusion regularization, the semi-implicit solution scheme, $\tau_1 = 1.0$ and $\alpha_1 = 0.5$, see 7.2.3.2), with the single exception that only the affine pre-registration step was performed. This is done because a nonlinear surface alignment would bias an evaluation based on the surface overlap.

Evaluating inter-patient registration is a challenging task because annotating corresponding landmarks in the images is impracticable. Therefore, matching was quantitatively evaluated considering $\mathcal{M}^{Dice}$ and $\mathcal{M}^{Mean}$ for the alignment of lung and lobe segmentations after registration.

Atlas generation To demonstrate the applicability of the registration framework for atlas generation, a mean intensity image was computed in a second study applying the iterative approach detailed in Section 7.2.4.2. This atlas is also used for initialization in Section 7.3.

For the registration, the symmetric diffeomorphic framework was employed with dual NSSD forces because the inverse transformation is required during the atlas generation process (see Section 7.2.4.2). As derived in Section 3.4, the inverse transformation can be computed very efficiently from the velocity field. Moreover, the average operation is properly defined for the group of diffeomorphisms and can be calculated efficiently using the velocity fields and exploiting the properties of the lie algebra. A more detailed explanation is given in [Ehrhardt et al. 2011].

The quality of the generated atlas was visually assessed.

7.2.4.2 Bias-free atlas generation

A mean intensity atlas was generated using the approach presented by Guimond et al. [1998]. First, the 9 images I_p of the training data pool with $p = 1, \ldots, 9$ were registered to one arbitrarily chosen reference image using the described registration approach, yielding the transformation $\varphi_j^{(0)}$. All images were then transformed to the reference frame by $I_p \circ \varphi_p^{(0)}$ and the mean image $\bar{I}^{(0)}$ was computed.

To avoid a bias due to the choice of the reference frame, an iterative procedure was pursued. For this, the mean transformation $\bar{\varphi}^{(0)}$ was computed and its inverse used to transform the mean image. In the next step, registration of all images was rerun with $\bar{I}^{(0)} \circ (\bar{\varphi}^{(0)})^{-1}$ as reference image. This procedure was repeated for n iterations until the average transformation converged against the identity and the mean shape and intensity atlas $\bar{I}^{(n)}$ was obtained.

To improve the results with regard to the application for segmentation initialization in Section 7.3, separate atlases were built for left and right lung.

7.2.4.3 Results

Pairwise registration The results show a precise alignment of the lungs after registration. On average, $\mathcal{M}^{Dice} = 0.99$ and $\mathcal{M}^{Mean} = 4.10$ mm is obtained. A comparably good alignment is not reached for the interlobular fissures. Here, the average Dice value is only $\mathcal{M}^{Dice} = 0.87$ and the according mean fissure distance $\mathcal{M}^{Mean} = 11.95$ mm (9.79 mm for left fissure, 14.72 mm for right horizontal fissure). The complete results are presented in Table 7.5 in the context of lobe alignment.

Atlas generation The generated atlas is visualized for both lungs in Figure 7.9 (left). A high contrast is visible indicating a proper alignment of the major airways. However, it cannot be ensured that only corresponding airways are aligned in every case. To this end, an anatomical annotation of the structures would be required.

7.2.5 Discussion

The results presented in this section substantiate a very high accuracy of the registration algorithm for intra-patient registration. For both the motion estimation in Section 7.2.2 as well as the EMPIRE10 study in Section 7.2.3, the landmark alignment error $\mathcal{M}^{LAE}$ lies in the dimension of the voxel spacing. Moreover, with values of 1.16 mm (WashU), 1.34 mm (DIR-lab) and 0.99 mm (POPI), the results are in the range of the best available approaches [Brock et al. 2010]. This was confirmed in the EMPIRE10 study [Murphy et al. 2011b].

A further advantage of the presented framework is its flexibility. As demonstrated in the studies, the components of the algorithm can be chosen to meet the specific requirements of the application (for example, standard vs. diffeomorphic approach, active vs. dual forces).

In the context of the EMPIRE10 study, a considerable dependence on the results of the pre-registration was apparent. In other words, optimizing the pre-registration is as important as optimizing the core algorithm. It can therefore be concluded that this step bears the potential for further improvement.

For inter-patient registration, evaluation could not be carried out with the same profoundness since no landmarks were available. However, quantitative results regarding $\mathcal{M}^{Dice}$ and $\mathcal{M}^{Mean}$ suggest a very precise alignment of the lung boundaries but a less accurate alignment of inner-lung structures. This is addressed in Section 7.4 by incorporating explicit fissure alignment in the registration algorithm.

Furthermore, the results show that it is imperative to consider lung physiology in the registration algorithm to preserve the discontinuous motion at the lung boundaries. In the section at hand, this was done using a masked registration, which does not yield a

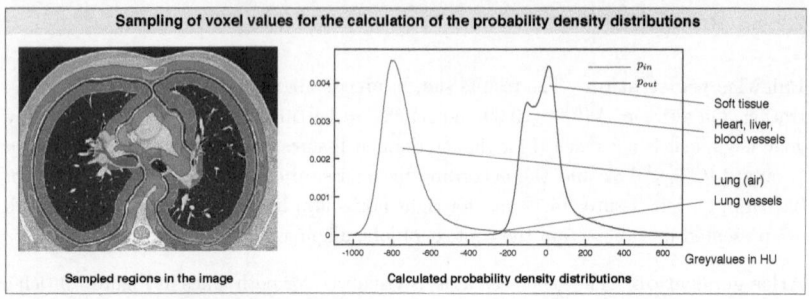

Figure 7.8: Left: regions inside (green) and outside (blue) the lung used for the sampling of the greyvalue distributions. On the right, p_{in} and p_{out} are given that result from the kernel density estimation on the sets of samples.

valid estimate of the background motion. This problem is addressed by applying the direction-dependent regularization in Section 7.5.

7.3 Evaluation of lobe segmentation with level sets

Before registration with integrated fissure alignment is analyzed, level set-based lobe segmentation is evaluated independently. The study described in the following is based on [Schmidt-Richberg et al. 2012d].

7.3.1 Estimation of greyvalue distributions

A precise estimation of the greyvalue probability distributions p_{in} (inside lung) and p_{out} (outside lung) is crucial for the region-based level set segmentation (4.4). Assuming that the distributions are similar for different scans of an image pool – which is very feasible because the greyvalues of CT images reflect the physically meaningful Houndsfield units of the respective tissue – they can be estimated using a set of segmented images and transferred to other images of that pool.

To this end, voxels are sampled in each image I with known reference segmentation S_I in a region inside and outside the object. The sets of samples are defined by

$$\mathcal{G}_{in} := \{I(\boldsymbol{x}_j) : \boldsymbol{x}_j \in \Omega^{\#} \wedge a_{in} \leq \text{dist}(\boldsymbol{x}_j, S_I) \leq b_{in}\}$$

and

$$\mathcal{G}_{out} := \{I(\boldsymbol{x}_j) : \boldsymbol{x}_j \in \Omega^{\#} \wedge a_{out} \leq \text{dist}(\boldsymbol{x}_j, S_I^{-1}) \leq b_{out}\},$$

with S_I^{-1} denoting the inverted segmentation, that means the background. The region for the sampling is determined with respect to the Euclidean distance $\text{dist}(\boldsymbol{x}_j, S_I)$

of the voxels $\boldsymbol{x}_j$ to the object boundary in S_I. Outer limits b_{in} and b_{out} are chosen depending on the anticipated accuracy of the initialization: If it is expected to be far apart from the object, a larger region has to be considered for the sampling. Inner limits $a_{in}, a_{out} > 0$ can be chosen to circumvent partial volume effects and inaccuracies of the reference segmentations. In this work, both intervals were set to $[a_{in/out}, b_{in/out}] := [3, 15]$.

Given the sampling sets $\mathcal{G}_{in/out} = \{g_1, \ldots, g_G\}$ with $G := |\mathcal{G}_{in/out}|$ being the sample size, the corresponding greyvalue probability density distributions p_{in} and p_{out} are assessed using a kernel density estimation following Parzen [1962] by

$$p_{in/out}(g) := \frac{1}{G} \sum_{j=1}^{G} \frac{1}{\sigma\sqrt{2\pi}} \exp\left(-0,5\frac{(g-g_j)^2}{\sigma^2}\right).$$

The approach is illustrated in Figure 7.8.

7.3.2 Atlas-based initialization of the segmentation

In this work, a coarse initialization was generated using an simplistic atlas-based segmentation approach. First, a mean intensity atlas was generated separately for each lung employing the iterative approach presented in Section 7.2.4.2. Using the transformations $\varphi_p^{(n)}$ computed in this context, the known reference segmentations S_{I_p} were transferred to the coordinate system of the atlas and then combined using the standard vote rule to represent a segmentation of the mean shape and intensity image [Aljabar et al. 2009]. An initialization for the segmentation of an unseen test image was then computed by registering that image to the atlas and transferring the atlas segmentation to the image.

It has to be noted that the atlas was not generated using a leave-one-our strategy but considering all images of the pool. This was done mainly for computational reasons. However, the atlas is only used for initialization and Ehrhardt et al. [2011] observed that minor variations of the data pool have only a small influence on the atlas. The introduced bias is therefore considered to be negligible.

The generated mean intensity atlas and corresponding segmentations of the pulmonary lobes are illustrated in Figure 7.9.

7.3.3 Study setup

Normal-dose data   The core evaluation is based on the RUKSH data set and the manual lobe segmentation generated for this purpose (see Section 7.1.2).

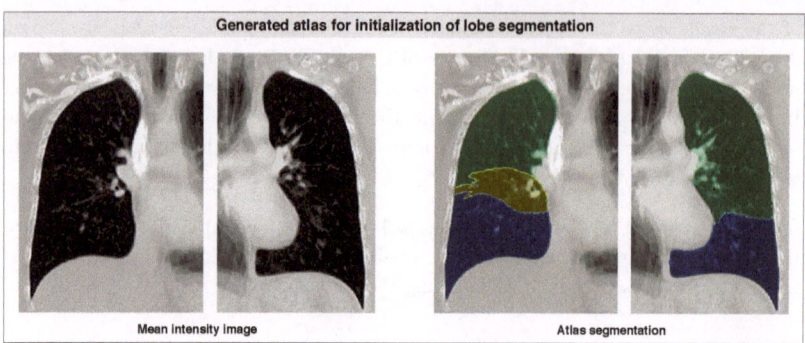

Figure 7.9: Left: The mean intensity atlas generated from the RUKSH image pool using the approach detailed in Section 7.2.4.2. Right: The lobe segmentation of the atlas generated by the vote rule using the transformed ground truth segmentations of the images.

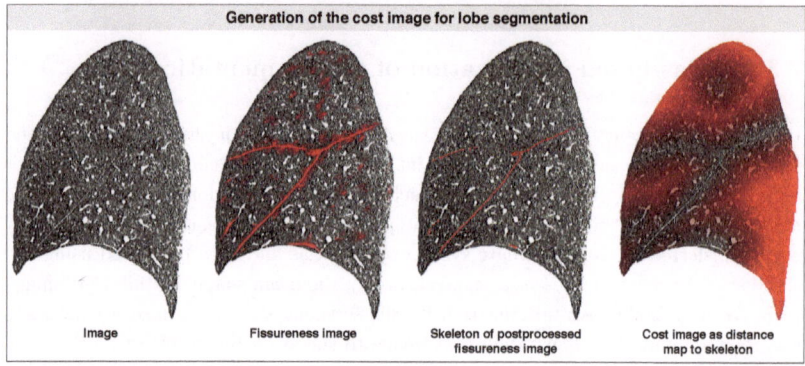

Figure 7.10: Steps for the computation of the cost image, from left to right: the CT image I; the fissureness image F, obtained as output of the $k$nn classifier; the skeleton K of the post-processed fissureness image (dilated by one voxel to enhance visibility); the cost image C, which is incorporated in the force term. [Modified from source: Schmidt-Richberg et al. 2012d]

First, a segmented atlas was generated using the whole image pool as described in the preceding section. In the next step, the greyvalue distributions were estimated for each image. To avoid a bias, a leave-one-out strategy was applied, that means for the segmentation of image I_p greyvalues were sampled in each image I_q with $p \neq q$. Similarly, 1000 fissure- and background voxels were sampled per image to train the classifier for fissure segmentation, resulting in 16k samples in total. All parameters (number k of nearest neighbors, selected features) were chosen as proposed in [van Rikxoort et al. 2008] and not optimized for the data pool. The cost images were computed according to Section 5.2.2.1 as illustrated in Figure 7.10.

Optimal parameters were empirically determined to be $\tau = 0.5$, $\alpha = 0.5$, $\gamma = 0.5$ and used unaltered for all images. A total of 600 iterations were performed on two resolution levels.

For each patient p, three segmentations S_p were compared with the manual reference segmentation M_p: the atlas-based initialization S_p^{Init}, the result S_p^{Std} of the standard multi-object level set segmentation (4.10) without the additional force term for lobe alignment and the result S_p^{Lobe} of the proposed lobe segmentation approach (5.4). As metrics, the Dice coefficient $\mathcal{M}^{Dice}$, the mean fissure distance $\mathcal{M}^{Mean}$ and the fissure alignment measure $\mathcal{M}^{Fiss}$ were considered.

Low-dose data   In a second evaluation experiment, the segmentation approach was exemplarily tested on low-dose CT scans from the EMPIRE10 pool. In particular, the reference images of the test cases 14, 20 and 21 were regarded to appraise the applicability of the segmentation algorithm in the integrated registration framework for enhanced fissure alignment. These pairs were chosen because a conspicuously bad performance in the fissure alignment category was observed for the majority of participating algorithms of the EMPIRE challenge [Murphy et al. 2011b].[3]

Two approaches were followed for initialization: On the one hand, the atlas generated from the RUKSH data was used as in the preceding experiments. On the other hand, the lobe segmentation of the template image was assumed to be known and used as initial segmentation after affine alignment. This procedure simulates the application in the integrated framework for fissure alignment (see Section 7.4).

Parameter values were chosen as above, but evaluation metrics are confined to $\mathcal{M}^{Mean}$ and $\mathcal{M}^{Fiss}$, which are considered to be more meaningful than the Dice coefficient.

7.3.4 Results

Normal-dose data   Exemplary results of the presented approach for lobe segmentation are shown for the RUKSH data in Figure 7.11. The atlas-based initialization (second column) depicts the approximate anatomy of the lungs but lobe boundaries are often remote from the actual fissures. Using the multi-object level set approach without additional force term (third column), lung boundaries are segmented precisely but in the inside of the lung only the smoothing condition applies. Adding the presented force term causes an attraction of the lobe boundaries to the fissures (last column). The strength of the approach becomes apparent in areas with gaps in the detected fissure segmentations: Due to the formulation of the cost image as distance map, the level set automatically finds the shortest connection between the fissure segments.

---

[3] The scan pair 28 is also characterized by a bad result in the fissure alignment category. However, fissures are barely visible and establishing a ground truth seemed arbitrary in this case. Therefore, it is refrained from regarding patient 28 in this work.

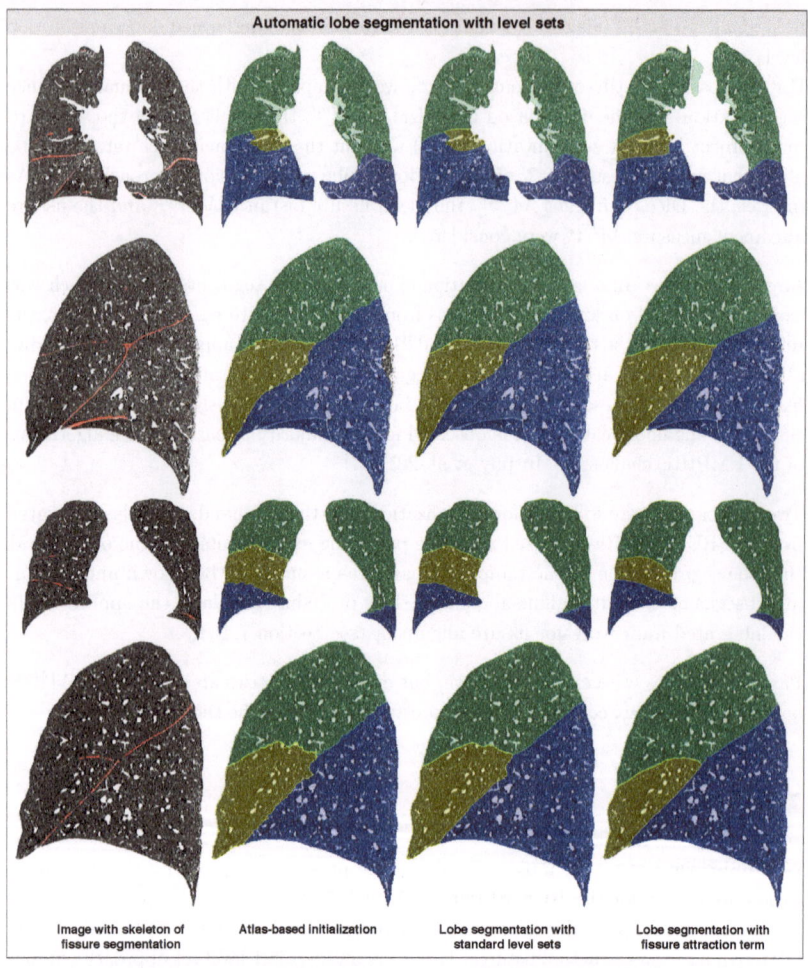

Figure 7.11: From left to right: a) the image I with the skeleton K of the fissure segmentation as red
overlay; b) the atlas-based initialization of the segmentation; c) the result of the standard
level set segmentation; d) the result of the level set segmentation with additional fissure
attraction force.

Quantitative results are given in Table 7.3. In all cases, lobe segmentations are
considerably enhanced using the presented fissure attraction force. The improvement
is also statistically significant ($p \leq 0.005$) for all metrics except the Dice coefficient of
the right superior and middle lobe. It is also apparent that left lobes are segmented
considerably better (mean fissure distance 1.74 mm) than the three right lobes (3.18
and 10.5 mm).

Table 7.3: Quantitative evaluation results for the three segmentations, averaged over all nine data sets: the initial segmentation S^{Init}, the standard level set segmentation S^{Std} and the level set segmentation with additional lobe force S^{Lobe}.

Metric	Lobe/Fissure	S^{Init}	S^{Std}	S^{Lobe}
$\mathcal{M}^{Dice}$	left superior	0.94 ± 0.02	0.94 ± 0.02	0.98 ± 0.00
	left inferior	0.94 ± 0.03	0.94 ± 0.02	0.98 ± 0.01
	right superior	0.93 ± 0.02	0.94 ± 0.02	0.97 ± 0.02
	right middle	0.78 ± 0.06	0.78 ± 0.06	0.83 ± 0.13
	right inferior	0.92 ± 0.02	0.92 ± 0.02	0.93 ± 0.06
	mean	0.90 ± 0.02	0.90 ± 0.02	0.94 ± 0.04
$\mathcal{M}^{Fiss}$	left	0.25 ± 0.22	0.24 ± 0.21	0.83 ± 0.07
	right oblique	0.25 ± 0.16	0.24 ± 0.16	0.76 ± 0.13
	right horizontal	0.24 ± 0.12	0.23 ± 0.12	0.48 ± 0.24
$\mathcal{M}^{Mean}$	left	8.56 ± 4.41	9.01 ± 4.55	1.74 ± 0.47
	right oblique	8.30 ± 2.93	8.99 ± 3.03	3.18 ± 2.95
	right horizontal	10.6 ± 5.73	11.5 ± 6.14	10.5 ± 9.48

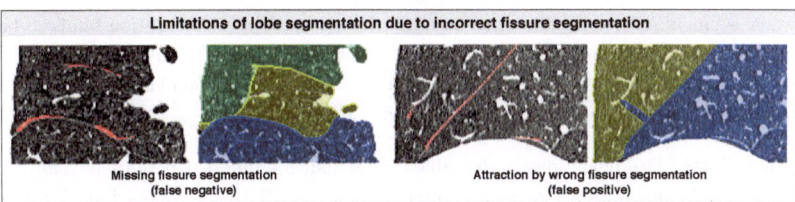

Limitations of lobe segmentation due to incorrect fissure segmentation

Missing fissure segmentation
(false negative)

Attraction by wrong fissure segmentation
(false positive)

Figure 7.12: Limitations of the presented approach: Incomplete fissure segmentations (left) or structures incorrectly classified as fissures (right) can impair the segmentation result.

Two aspects of the algorithm emerged as crucial for the segmentation quality: the calculation of the cost image and the initialization. Fissure segmentation is sensitive to image quality and may therefore be insufficient for images with low resolution or reconstruction artifacts. While gaps in the fissures can be compensated by the level set formulation, the segmentation might be impaired if a whole part of a fissure is missing. This is demonstrated in Figure 7.12 (left), where the boundary is attracted by the oblique fissure because the horizontal fissure is detected incompletely. The inverse problem is caused if structures are falsely classified as fissure and therefore attract the segmentation (Figure 7.12, right). These limitations are evident especially in areas where the initialization is unsatisfying and apart from the fissures. Here, the segmentation may be attracted either by the wrong fissure or by other structures or noise in the images falsely classified as fissures.

Low-dose data The presented segmentation algorithm does not achieve the same accuracy for the EMPIRE10 data as for the RUKSH data, as shown in Table 7.4. Due to

Table 7.4: Quantitative evaluation results for the EMPIRE data, averaged over the three regarded data sets. The initial segmentation S^{Init} is compared to the level set segmentation with additional lobe force S^{Lobe}. Two approaches for initialization are regarded: On the one hand, the same atlas-based initialization as for the normal-dose data, on the other hand an initialization based on another time point of the 4D data set.

Metric	Lobe/Fissure	Init.: Atlas S^{Init}	S^{Lobe}	Init.: Template Seg. S^{Init}	S^{Lobe}
$\mathcal{M}^{Fiss}$	left	0.08 ± 0.02	0.66 ± 0.12	0.11 ± 0.07	0.72 ± 0.10
	right oblique	0.10 ± 0.10	0.60 ± 0.12	0.18 ± 0.15	0.70 ± 0.06
	right horizontal	0.08 ± 0.01	0.30 ± 0.03	0.54 ± 0.11	0.58 ± 0.17
$\mathcal{M}^{Mean}$	left	9.28 ± 1.17	3.17 ± 2.11	6.74 ± 2.56	1.92 ± 0.53
	right oblique	11.3 ± 7.75	5.06 ± 2.57	7.56 ± 3.13	3.72 ± 2.04
	right horizontal	11.0 ± 2.07	9.52 ± 3.34	5.01 ± 2.64	5.75 ± 2.30

the lower image quality and in particular the lower resolution, fissure detection is prone to misclassification caused by noise. This has crucial influence on the lobe segmentation as it increases the risk of misleading attraction forces. As revealed by a considerably worse segmentation using the atlas-based initialization, lobe segmentation tends to be attracted by structures falsely classified as fissures. Using an initialization based on the segmentation of the template image, however, the initial lobe boundaries are closer to the detected fissures and the algorithm yields satisfying results.

The high standard deviations in the table further indicate different performance for the data sets. While lobes are segmented precisely for case 21 (intra-patient initialization: $\mathcal{M}^{Fiss} = 0.76$ averaged over all fissures), quality is considerably worse for case 20 ($\mathcal{M}^{Fiss} = 0.62$). This further stresses the importance of a performant initialization and fissure detection.

Confirming the observations made above, the results again show a higher segmentation precision for the left lung, while in particular the right oblique fissure is segmented with poor quality.

7.3.5 Discussion

The evaluation study presented in this section reveals a generally high accuracy of the level-set based approach for lobe segmentation using normal-dose CT images. The method performs best for the left lung where on average a proportion of 83% of the interlobular fissure was precisely aligned. In the right lung, only 76% and 48% of oblique and horizontal fissure were traced correctly. This is explained by the risk of the level set being attracted by the wrong fissure if the initialization is considerably apart. Moreover, detection of the right horizontal fissure is often inferior to the other two fissures.

Using the same atlas-based initialization approach for the low-dose data of the EM-PIRE10 pool, no comparable accuracy was reached. Due to the poor image quality and lower resolution, fissure detection is susceptible for misclassifications, which cause the segmentation to be attracted by the wrong structures. However, this is compensated using a better initialization, which can be provided by intra-patient registration if the segmentation of the template image is known. This is of relevance in the joint registration framework for fissure alignment.

To further improve accuracy, several approaches can be followed. First, a more accurate detection of the fissures would imply an eminent benefit – in particular for the low-dose data, for which fissures were segmented insufficiently. To this end, a more thorough and especially data-specific optimization of the parameters for $k$nn classification is particularly promising [van Rikxoort et al. 2008]. Moreover, a more sophisticated post-processing of the fissureness image bears the potential for further improvement.
Second, the results show that the method depends on a reasonably good initialization. This could be provided using advanced multi-atlas techniques, which are primarily investigated for brain imaging in current literature [Wolz et al. 2010].
Third, additional anatomical information could be considered in the approach. For example, Ukil and Reinhardt [2009], van Rikxoort et al. [2010] or Doel et al. [2012] use airways and vessel tree for a coarse orientation of the fissures. This information could either be incorporated in the initialization step or as an additional pushing term in the level set framework.

In summary, the presented method is capable of sufficiently well aligning the pulmonary lobes, even though current methods with the sole purpose of lobe segmentation are probably superior, in particular for low-dose data (see Section 5.2.1). This should be validated in further studies by directly comparing different algorithms on the same image base. However, aiming for improved fissure alignment for lung registration, results are very promising and the variational formulation of the approach enables an integration with the registration.

7.4 Evaluation of registration with fissure alignment

An evaluation of the combined segmentation and registration approach for increased fissure alignment is in the focus of the section at hand. The results presented in the following cover and extend the findings published in [Schmidt-Richberg et al. 2012b].

7.4.1 Study setup

Inter-patient registration for atlas generation As for the lobe segmentation algorithm, core evaluation is based on the RUKSH image pool. To avoid a bias by the choice of the reference image, a pairwise validation was employed, that means each image was registered with the remaining eight images, leading to 72 registrations.

As registration components, the standard approach with masked active NSSD forces, diffusion regularization and the semi-implicit solution scheme were chosen in accordance with Section 7.2.4 ($\tau_1 = 1.0$, $\alpha_1 = 0.5$, four resolution scales). The segmentation parameters were chosen as specified in Section 7.3 ($\tau_2 = 0.5$, $\alpha_2 = 1.0$, $\gamma = 0.5$). The values of the additional parameters $\beta_1 = 0.5$ and $\beta_2 = 0.1$ were determined by an empiric optimization process. Since the segmentation converges faster than the registration, five registration iterations were performed for each segmentation iteration.

For a quantitative evaluation, the transformation computed with the common registration approach minimizing $\mathcal{J}^{Reg}$ was compared to the presented registration with integrated lobe segmentation $\mathcal{J}^{Joint}$. As metrics, the $\mathcal{M}^{Dice}$, the mean fissure distance $\mathcal{M}^{Mean}$ and the fissure alignment measure $\mathcal{M}^{Fiss}$ of the manual reference segmentation S_R and transformed template segmentation $S_T \circ \varphi$ were considered. Furthermore, the Dice coefficient and the mean surface distance of the lung were assessed to quantify lung alignment.

Intra-patient registration for motion estimation In a second study, the test cases 14, 20 and 21 of the EMPIRE10 pool were regarded in accordance with Section 7.3. Segmentation and registration parameters were chosen as above.

7.4.2 Results

Inter-patient registration Quantitative results for the RUKSH data are given in Table 7.5. For the joint approach, they exhibit a significantly better alignment of the lung boundaries than for the standard registration by reducing the mean surface distance from 4.10 mm to 3.07 mm ($p \leq 0.001$). Results further confirm a significantly better alignment of the lung fissures using the proposed registration approach ($p \leq 0.05$ for all metrics and subjects serving as reference image). Averaged over all registrations, 40% of the fissures are well aligned using the joint approach, compared to only 16% with the standard method. The mean distance is reduced from 12.0 mm to 7.8 mm. Results are better for the left lung (52%) than for the fissures in the right lung (44% and 24% for horizontal and oblique fissures). The same observations hold for the mean fissure distance.

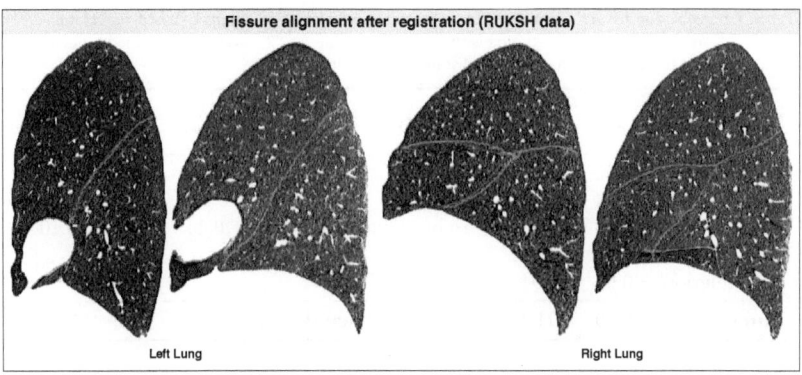

Figure 7.13: Reference images with lobe boundaries as color overlay. Red: manual reference segmentation; Blue: template segmentation after registration with $\mathcal{J}^{Reg}$; Green: template segmentation after registration with $\mathcal{J}^{Joint}$. In most regions of the image, fissure alignment is considerably improved using the integrated approach. However, in regions with missing sections in the detected fissures – in particular close to the lung boundaries – no improvement is achieved. This is observed mainly in the right lung, for which fissure detection is more challenging.

The results are visualized in Figure 7.13. A much better alignment of the fissures is apparent in regions where fissures were segmented successfully. Furthermore, in a proof-of-concept demonstration the application to atlas generation is explored and illustrated in Figure 7.14. Here, lobe segmentations of eight subjects were transformed to the remaining subject and averaged. The joint registration approach provides a much sharper segmentation of the reference image, which indicates an improved matching of the lobes.

In total, computation time lies between 6 min and 14 min, which implies a prolongation of approximately 48% in comparison to the standard registration.

Intra-patient registration   As for the normal-dose data, lung alignment is considerably improved by integration of the segmentation. On average, the mean surface distance $\mathcal{M}^{Mean}$ was reduced from 0.24 mm to 0.05 mm.

Since lobe segmentation is considerably more challenging for the low-dose data, registration with explicit fissure alignment did not entail the same improvement for the EMPIRE10 data as for the RUKSH data. In particular, differences between the cases are apparent. While the mean fissure distance $\mathcal{M}^{Mean}$ was reduced from on average 3.07 mm to 2.19 mm for case 21, the metric only changed from 4.00 mm to 3.68 mm for case 20. Case 14 yields an average result with an improvement from 4.07 mm to 3.40 mm.

Table 7.5: Lobe and fissure alignment after registration with common intensity-based registration $\mathcal{J}^{Reg}$ and the proposed registration with fissure alignment $\mathcal{J}^{Joint}$, averaged over the results of all 72 image pairs. The mean fissure distance is given in millimeter.

Lobe	$\mathcal{M}^{Dice}$		Fissure	$\mathcal{M}^{Fiss}$		$\mathcal{M}^{Mean}$	
	$\mathcal{J}^{Reg}$	$\mathcal{J}^{Joint}$		$\mathcal{J}^{Reg}$	$\mathcal{J}^{Joint}$	$\mathcal{J}^{Reg}$	$\mathcal{J}^{Joint}$
left superior	0.92	0.95	left	0.18	0.52	9.79	4.74
left inferior	0.93	0.95					
right superior	0.88	0.90	right oblique	0.16	0.44	11.34	6.10
right middle	0.69	0.73	right horizontal	0.15	0.24	14.72	12.70
right inferior	0.91	0.94					
Lung	0.99	0.99	**Mean surface distance**			4.10	3.07

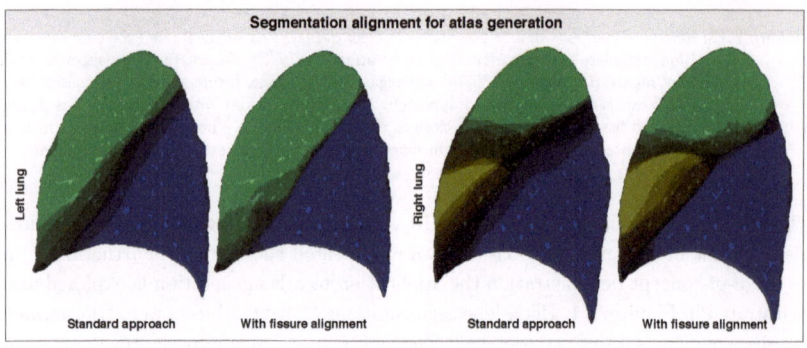

Figure 7.14: For this study, eight patients were registered with the remaining subject. Afterwards, the lobe segmentations of each subject were transformed to the domain of the reference image and averaged. The joint approach with explicit fissure alignment produces a sharper and therefore more consistent atlas segmentation than the standard registration.

7.4.3 Discussion

The results demonstrate that integrating lobe information in intensity-based registration can improve fissure alignment considerably. Employing level set methods to this end entails several advantages over – for example – directly considering the cost image C. First, forces are only generated along the zero level set, that means only at the fissures and not at places wrongly classified as fissures due to noise. Gaps in the fissure segmentations are not exceedingly critical since they are automatically bridged by the level set framework. If no fissure information is present in an image region, no forces (besides smoothing) are generated that move ϕ_R away from ϕ_T and thus only the standard registration is applied in this area. This effect could be enhanced by truncating C to restrain the influence of the fissure alignment to a smaller range, for example if segmentation is suffering from bad image quality.

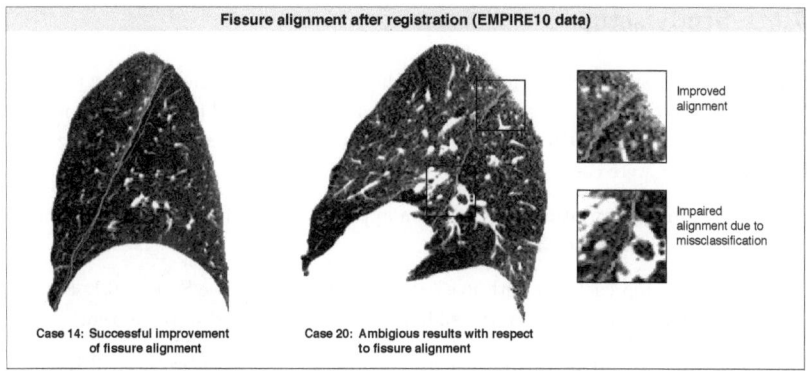

Figure 7.15: Fissure alignment for motion estimation using the EMPIRE10 data. Red: manual reference segmentation; Blue: template segmentation after registration with $\mathcal{J}^{Reg}$; Green: template segmentation after registration with $\mathcal{J}^{Joint}$. For test case 14 the fissure distance is slightly reduced in the whole image. However, for case 20 fissure detection is erroneous due to the low image quality. For this patient, some regions show an improvement while an aggravation of the misalignment is observed in other regions.

Naturally, the benefit of the presented method depends on the segmentation quality. For the lung boundaries, which can be segmented particularly robust, a significantly enhanced alignment is observed for all considered images. Since fissure segmentation is far more challenging, results vary depending on the image quality. This is especially notable regarding the EMPIRE10 data, for which results are less accurate than for the RUKSH pool.

Problems arise in particular in the right lung between horizontal and oblique fissures because the fissure enhancement filter performs worse in this region. Moreover, the level set can be attracted by the wrong fissure if the initialization is insufficient. A more precise initialization – for example using an anatomical atlas – could improve the results in this area.

7.5 Evaluation of motion estimation with direction-dependent regularization

The last section of this chapter is targeted at an evaluation of the presented direction-dependent regularization approach. The results combine the findings presented in [Schmidt-Richberg et al. 2012a] and [Schmidt-Richberg et al. 2012e].

7.5.1 Study setup

The focus of this study lies on an analysis of the impact of sliding motion on registration-based motion estimation. All referred 4D data sets are considered for evaluation, namely WashU, DIR-lab and POPI. To assess the benefit of sliding-preserving regularization, four approaches were compared to each other:

A1   The standard variational registration approach with diffusion regularization as presented in Chapter 3.

A2   The same approach but with masked force computation, see Section 6.1. For this method, a segmentation of the sliding object was assumed to be known.

A3   The basic direction-dependent regularization presented in Section 6.2.1, which equally relies on a segmentation of the object.

A4   The direction-dependent regularization with automatic detection of sliding motion as described in Sect. 6.2.2, for which no segmentation is required.

Moreover, the benefit of FED over the explicit solution scheme was analyzed. In analogy to Section 7.2.2, a second registration run was performed, in which computation time was limited to 10 (DIR-lab, POPI) or 15 minutes (WashU) per data set. To judge the results it should be noted that one iteration with DDR takes approximately 35% longer than with diffusion regularization, resulting in considerably less iterations. Apart from that, the standard non-diffeomorphic framework with passive NSSD forces was used consistently in all experiments.

A multi-resolution strategy with 4 levels was applied in all runs. The values of step size and regularization weight have been chosen as determined in Section 7.2.2 ($\alpha = 0.07$, explicit scheme: $\tau = 0.2$, FED: $T = 5.0$). The parameters of the weighting functions employed in A3 and A4 were left unaltered for all data sets and experiments showed that the algorithm is very robust to their choice. Applied values are $c_1 = 200$, $c_2 = 1$ in (6.3) and $c_1 = 3$, $c_2 = 8$ in (6.7).

For a quantitative evaluation of the registration results, accuracy is quantified as landmark alignment error $\mathcal{M}^{LAE}$.

7.5.2 Results

Qualitative comparison   In Figure 7.16, a qualitative comparison of the four regularization approaches is shown. While the motion fields are very similar around the bronchial tree, considerable differences occur close to the outer lung boundaries. Using the standard regularization approach A1, motion vectors are smoothed comprehensively between object and background. As a result, the (upwards moving) background has a huge impact on the (downwards moving) object, which leads to an underestimation of

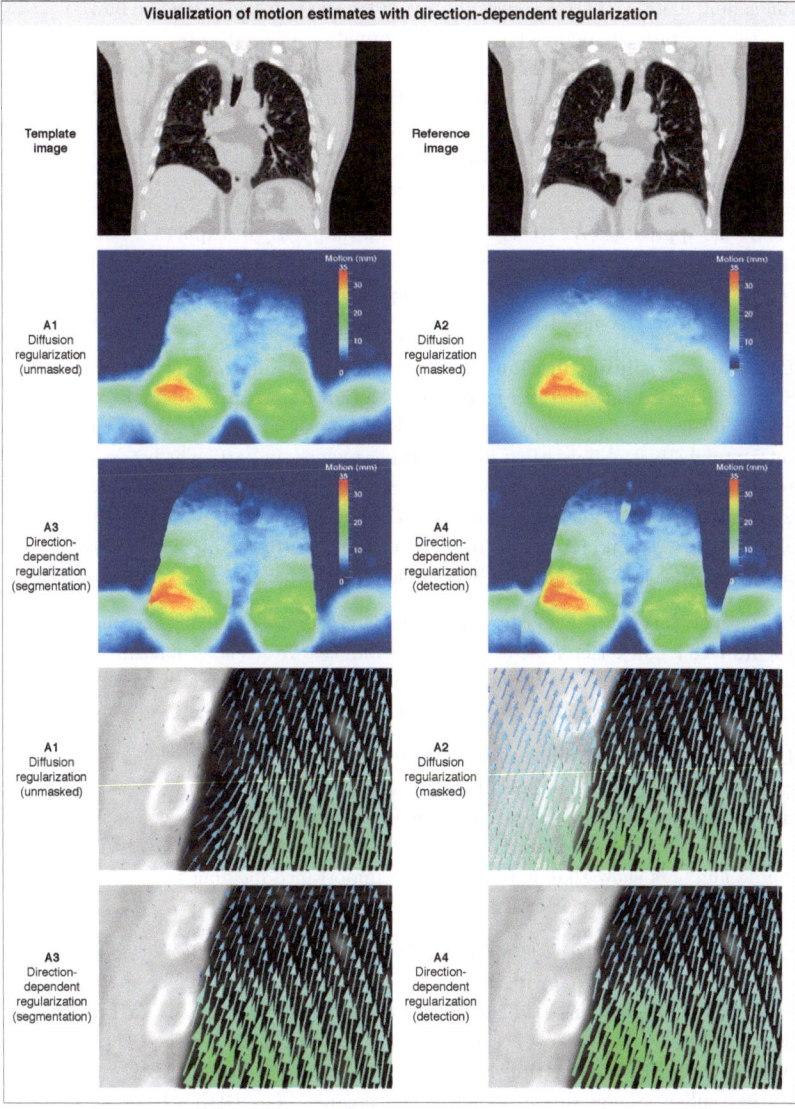

Figure 7.16: Visualization of registration results for one patient of the WashU data pool. Top: template (left) and reference image (right). Below: results for unmasked (A1) and masked (A2) registration, DDR with segmentation (A3) and detection of discontinuous motion (A4). The estimation using A2 is valid only inside the lung, motion vectors outside solely occur due to smoothing. [Modified from source: Schmidt-Richberg et al. 2012e]

inner lung motion. This is especially severe for the registration of the lungs because the rib cage provides detailed greyvalue information while the inner lung is relatively homogeneous (see Figure 7.17). In algorithm A2, this problem is implicitly avoided by masking the background and thus preventing it from influencing the registration. In comparison to A1, the motion estimated by the direction-dependent approaches A3 and A4 also much better satisfies the expectation derived from respiration physiology because sliding motion is clearly visible close to the lung boundaries.

While the approaches A2 to A4 are all able to (implicitly or explicitly) handle sliding motion and to improve the registration accuracy, the deformation field of the masked registration A2 is only valid inside the lungs. The direction-dependent approaches are qualitatively very similar to each other.

Detection of sliding motion   The detection of sliding motion as introduced in Section 6.2.2 is visualized in Figure 7.18. Motion is correctly assessed to be sliding at the pleurae along the rib cage and to be less sliding at the mediastinal region. Interestingly, it is also detected in some other regions, in particular between skin and background. While the correctness of this finding is unclear from a physical point of view, it is beneficial for the algorithm as the background will remain fixed when the skin moves. Also, no error is introduced to the registration of the skin because the background features no intensity information besides noise.

In contrast, image artifacts can impair the detection as seen along the diaphragm in Figure 7.18 (right). Here, the detection of candidate voxels is insufficient because the edge is blurred due to notable motion artifacts. Moreover, at voxels that were detected as candidates, the motion is wrongly rated as not sliding.

Landmark-based evaluation   Quantitative results of the landmark-based evaluation can be found in table 7.6. For all images, masked registration and registration with direction-dependent regularization yield better results than the common diffusion approach. This improvement is statistically significant (significance level $p \leq 0.05$). These numbers show that it is of eminent importance for lung registration to take motion physiology into account.

Comparing the solution schemes, FED yields significantly ($p \leq 0.05$) better results than the simple explicit scheme with fixed step sizes. This holds for all four approaches and confirms the observations made in Section 7.2.2. All together, the masked registration with FED results in the most accurate registration, closely followed by the combination of DDR with FED. In the time-limited second registration run, FED is still superior to the explicit scheme due to its faster convergence. The DDR/FED approach also outperforms unmasked diffusion regularization but the improvement is less prominent since computation is stopped before full convergence.

To further specify the benefit of the direction-dependent regularization, the landmark alignment error is analyzed subject to the distance of each landmark to the outer

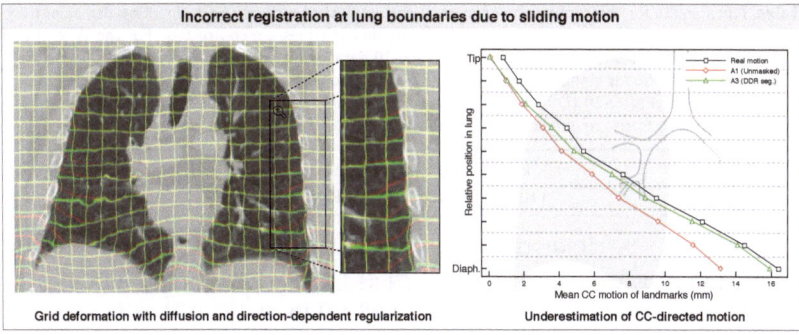

Figure 7.17: Left: The registration results visualized as transformed grid overlay for unmasked diffusion (red) and direction-dependent regularization (green). The influence of the registration of high-contrast rib cage to the low-contrast inner lung is particularly severe for diffusion regularization. Right: motion of landmarks in cranio-caudal direction subject to their relative position between tip of the lung and diaphragm, averaged over all patients. The unmasked registration leads to an underestimation of the motion due to the global smoothing. This problem increases with the motion amplitude – that is in caudal direction – and results in a difference between real motion and motion estimated by A1 of more than 3.0 mm near the diaphragm. This is successfully addressed by the direction-dependent regularization. [Modified from source: Schmidt-Richberg et al. 2012e]

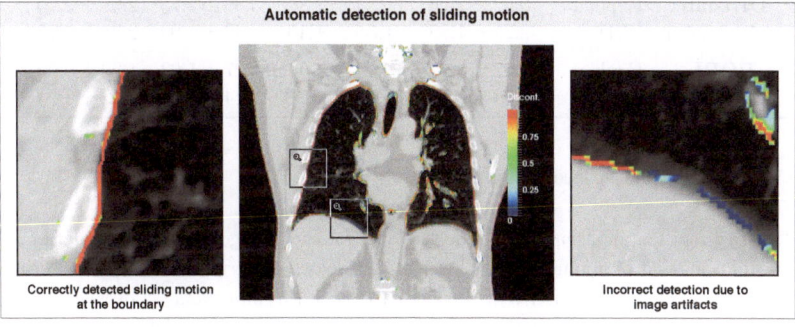

Figure 7.18: Visualization of the detected sliding motion as quantified by (6.7) for the same patient as in Figure 7.16. At red edges, discontinuous motion is detected, that means ω is close to 1. Blue points are candidate voxels that are rated to not feature sliding motion. [Modified from source: Schmidt-Richberg et al. 2012e]

lung boundary. On average, this distance is around 22.8 mm for all landmarks and patients. Considering only outliers of an unmasked registration, the distance is 13.6 mm, which shows that the most severe errors occur near the lung surface. This problem is successfully addressed by the direction-dependent regularization, as shown in Figure 7.19 where the improvement of algorithms A3 and A4 over A1 is plotted against the surface distance. The most significant improvement is observed in a region of around

Table 7.6: Results for the comparison of masked and unmasked diffusion with direction-dependent regularizers. Moreover, explicit and FED solution schemes are contrasted. For the WashU and DIR-lab data, the average over all 12 and 10 data sets is given. In the upper part of the table, registration is stopped only by the MSD-based stop criterion. In the lower part, registration is stopped after 10 (DIR-lab, POPI) and 15 (WashU) minutes, respectively. In contrast to 7.1, passive forces are employed. For the DIR-lab data, results are detailed in Appendix C.

Dataset (No reg.)	Scheme	Diffusion (unmasked)	Diffusion (masked)	DDR (seg.)	DDR (detect)
\- REGISTRATION UNTIL CONVERGENCE \-					
WashU	Explicit	1.78 ± 0.47	1.34 ± 0.23	1.43 ± 0.29	1.49 ± 0.42
(6.59 ± 1.78)	FED	1.74 ± 0.47	$\mathbf{1.28 \pm 0.18}$	1.33 ± 0.22	1.42 ± 0.38
DIR-lab	Explicit	3.05 ± 1.90	1.72 ± 0.47	2.13 ± 1.00	2.11 ± 0.91
(8.46 ± 3.33)	FED	2.91 ± 1.84	$\mathbf{1.51 \pm 0.30}$	1.71 ± 0.55	1.94 ± 0.84
POPI	Explicit	1.27	1.06	1.10	1.11
(7.15)	FED	1.22	$\mathbf{1.02}$	1.02	1.03
\- REGISTRATION FOR 10 (DIR-LAB, POPI) OR 15 (WASHU) MINUTES \-					
WashU	Explicit	1.80 ± 1.84	1.74 ± 1.86	1.84 ± 1.86	1.79 ± 1.87
(6.59 ± 4.49)	FED	1.48 ± 1.28	$\mathbf{1.31 \pm 0.95}$	1.60 ± 1.33	1.53 ± 1.15
DIR-lab	Explicit	3.02 ± 2.79	2.91 ± 2.88	3.08 ± 2.75	2.98 ± 2.75
(8.46 ± 5.48)	FED	2.22 ± 1.89	$\mathbf{1.55 \pm 1.11}$	2.49 ± 1.99	2.28 ± 1.73
POPI	Explicit	1.27 ± 1.02	1.21 ± 0.98	1.27 ± 1.02	1.22 ± 0.99
(7.15 ± 13.0)	FED	1.14 ± 0.55	$\mathbf{1.02 \pm 0.29}$	1.14 ± 0.55	1.02 ± 0.29

15.0 mm along the surface.

To assess registration accuracy outside the lung, for each image in the WashU data pool an additional set of about 20 outer-lung landmarks was determined along the rib cage. In this region, the LAE after registration with A1 is 1.55 mm averaged over all images (was 2.54 mm before registration). As visualized in Figure 7.20 (left), severe errors occur in particular at the ribs where the adjacent lung has a large motion amplitude. This is addressed by the direction-dependent regularization A3 (right, explicit scheme, average LAE 1.32 mm) and A4 (1.35 mm). The result of the masked registration A2 is not valid outside the lung (4.99 mm). This can be addressed by using an inverted mask and combining the fields (1.49 mm).

Lobe sliding As derived in Section 6.2.3, direction-dependent regularization can be extended in a straightforward manner to model sliding motion between multiple objects, for example the pulmonary lobes. This is exemplarily tested for one image of the WashU pool in a proof-of-concept evaluation. A lobe segmentation of the reference image was manually generated for this purpose.

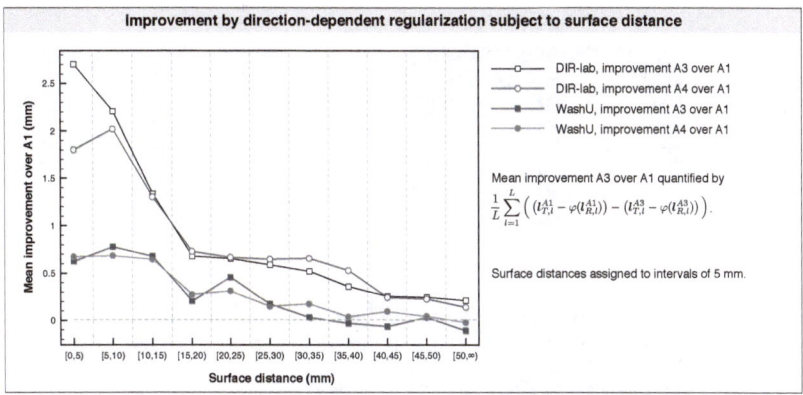

Figure 7.19: Improvement of A3 and A4 over A1 for the DIR-lab and the proprietary data. For each landmark, the improvement was quantified as misplacement with A1 minus error with A3/A4 and then averaged over all landmarks and patients separately for each distance interval. As the graph shows, the improvement is especially significant in a region of around 15 mm along the surface. [Modified from source: Schmidt-Richberg et al. 2012e]

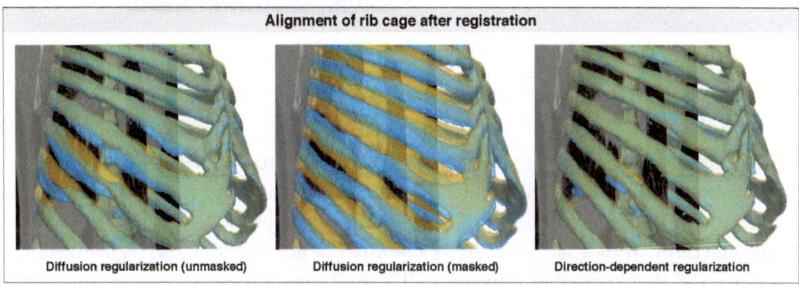

Figure 7.20: Segmentation of the rib cage of the reference image (orange) and of the target image (blue) after deformation with the result of unmasked (left, A1) masked (center, A2) and direction-dependent registration (right, A3). With unmasked registration, considerable errors occur due to the adjacent lung. The masked registration is not valid outside the lung. Only registration with direction-dependent regularization yields a satisfying result in the area of the rib cage. [Modified from source: Schmidt-Richberg et al. 2012e]

The resulting displacement field is illustrated in Figure 7.21 and compared with the computed field using a simple lung mask. Differences between the approaches are barely visible. However, by computing the difference field between the displacements, sliding motion becomes apparent at the boundary between two lobes. The landmark alignment error $\mathcal{M}^{LAE}$ is not noticeably improved because differences are small and no landmarks are in the proximity of the lobe boundaries.

Visual inspection further reveals that artifacts arise in regions where two lobes meet the lung boundary. This has several reasons. First, surface normals of neighboring

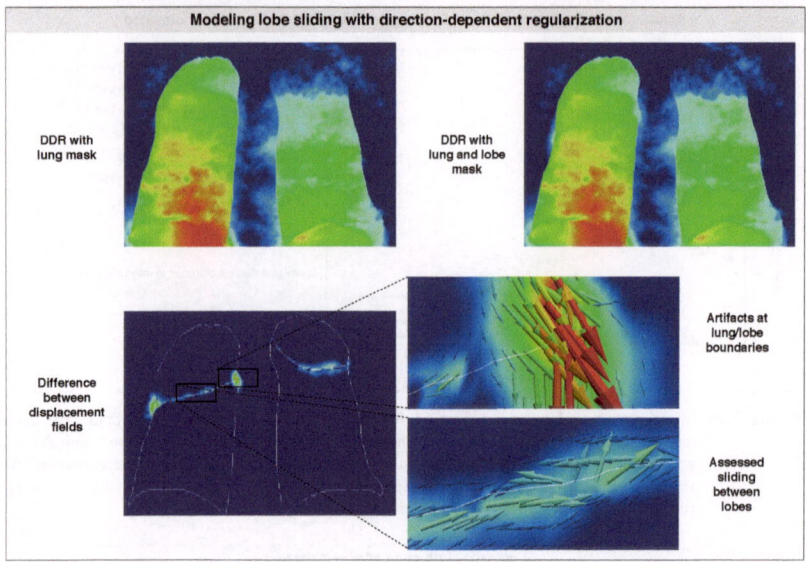

Figure 7.21: Distinctions between DDR with lung and lobe masks can only be made when regarding the difference field. Here, sliding motion is apparent between the individual lobes. However, artifacts arise at triple junctures, where two lobes meet the lung boundary.

objects do not differ only by the sign at triple junctures, that means they are not directly opposing. Second, the normal field is not smooth in this region, which violates the assumptions made in Section 6.2.1. Finally, segmentations can get very thin at triple junctures. If they have a width of one voxel in any direction, no regularization is performed in that particular dimension. To avoid these problems, an adaption of the model would be required.

7.5.3 Discussion

The study presented in this section illustrates the immense importance of considering breathing physiology in registration-based motion estimation. Incorporating knowledge about the sliding characteristics of the motion by either masking registration or applying direction-dependent regularization yields significantly better results than the standard approach.

Both variants of the direction-dependent regularization were compared. The segmentation-based method A3 slightly outperforms the approach A4 with automatic detection of sliding motion. This is mainly explained by artifacts in the images that impair motion sampling. In general, however, the assumptions on the characteristics of motion physiology made in Section 6.2.2 have been shown to be feasible to model sliding at lung boundaries. In other applications – for example to model sliding at the lung fissures – a candidate detection using the Deriche edge detector and a computation of object normals based on image gradients is not applicable. The same holds true for images from more noise-affected modalities like 4D MR or organs like the liver, which have been shown to feature sliding motion as well [Ding et al. 2009] but are low-contrasted in 4D CT. While the presented approach could principally be applied in a straightforward manner, candidate voxels and normals would have to be calculated in a different manner [Schmidt-Richberg et al. 2010b].

In general, masked registration (A2) performs slightly better than the direction-dependent approaches. However, the latter allow a closed mathematical formulation and a valid transformation is computed on the whole image domain, not only inside the mask. This is for example required to analyze correlation between skin and tumor motion for radiotherapy.

Naturally, computation time varies considerably depending on image size, number of iterations and the hardware used. While masking the images (A1) slightly decreases computation time per iteration, the direction-dependent approach A3 takes about 25% longer. Since the detection of sliding motion as described in A4 is done in every iteration, computation time is approximately doubled. However, the current implementation of this part would greatly benefit from runtime optimizations like parallelization.

Confirming the results of Section 7.2.2, FED significantly outperforms the explicit scheme for all considered approaches and should therefore always be employed. Still, exploring the possibilities to define a semi-implicit scheme would be of interest.

By modeling sliding motion between the pulmonary lobes, no improvement was achieved with respect to the landmark alignment error. This has several reasons. First, artifacts arise at triple junctures and impair the registration results. It is further questionable, if, on the one hand, image quality of the 4D data is sufficient to reliably assess lobe sliding and, on the other hand, lobe sliding plays a significant role during lung motion. While [Yin et al. 2010; Amelon et al. 2012] report considerable sliding between the lobes, underlying image data was acquired at breath-hold close to total lung capacity and not in the interval of natural breathing motion.

In summary, it is stated that motion physiology has to be addressed in the registration model if sliding motion occurs. The decision between masked or direction-dependent regularization should be done considering the specific requirements of the application.

Chapter 8

Conclusions

A precise registration of CT images of the lung is of eminent importance for various applications in pulmonary image analysis. The aim of this thesis has been to investigate how registration can benefit from an explicit consideration of lung-specific morphological and physiological characteristics. In detail, methods were developed to accurately align the pulmonary lobes and to model sliding motion at the lung boundaries. For both purposes, anatomical knowledge is incorporated based on a segmentation of the structure in demand.

In this chapter, the main contributions of this thesis are summarized. Moreover, perspectives are presented to point out possibilities for subsequent research projects.

8.1 Contributions

Three main contributions were made with this work. First, a general registration framework was formulated and optimized for intra- and inter-patient registration of lung CT scans. Second and third, two extensions for lobe alignment and modeling sliding motion were developed based on this framework. These contributions are summarized in the following.

Problem-specific optimization of a general registration approach　Inspired by current methods for lung registration, a flexible registration framework was formulated in Chapter 3. The modular design of the framework allows to customize the method for a specific task by adapting its main components, the similarity measure and the regularizer. Moreover, a possibility to restrain the transformation to the domain of diffeomorphisms was provided to enhance the plausibility of the transformation. To find a solution of the resulting registration problem, calculus of variations was employed with explicit, semi-implicit and Fast Explicit Diffusion schemes to solve the resulting Euler-Lagrange equations.

Extensive evaluation studies based on clinical CT data were provided in Section 7.2 to compare the different modules with application to lung registration. In detail, motion estimation based on 4D data, general intra-patient registration (for example, for baseline/follow-up examinations) as well as inter-patient registration were analyzed. In this context, the modular design turned out to be a major advantage as it allows to particularly address task-specific requirements like symmetry and invertibility. The key findings of the studies can be summarized as follows:

- The consideration of lung physiology is essential to account for the discontinuous motion at the lung boundaries. In the basic algorithm, this was done by restraining the registration to the inner-lung region using lung masks.

- NSSD forces significantly outperform standard SSD forces due to a better alignment of low-contrast regions such as the vasculature. Between the different NSSD formulations, only minor differences were identified with respect to registration accuracy.

- Elastic and diffusion regularization perform similarly well with the latter entailing computational benefits.

- The diffeomorphic approach entails a minor decrease in accuracy. However, foldings or singularities are obviated in the computed motion field, which indicates a more plausible transformation. Moreover, direct accessibility of the inverse transformation is particularly beneficial for atlas generation techniques.

- The semi-implicit solution scheme significantly outperforms the explicit scheme. It is also slightly superior to the Fast Explicit Diffusion, which on the other hand converges faster and may be advantageous in scenarios with limited computation time.

Furthermore, the results were submitted to the international EMPIRE10 study for intra-patient registration of the lung, in which a fourth place in a field of initially 34 participants was achieved [Murphy et al. 2011b]. This demonstrates that the developed algorithm is competitive with state-of-the-art methods.

Alignment of the pulmonary lobes The EMPIRE10 study revealed that the pulmonary lobes are often not well-aligned after registration with current algorithms. For inter-subject registration, this problem is considerably aggravated because anatomical differences between the patients have to be overcome. To address this, the approach followed in this work was motivated by the observations made in [Schmidt-Richberg et al. 2009c], which demonstrated exemplarily for the liver that a consideration of morphological knowledge can considerably improve the registration. With this in mind, a joint registration and segmentation approach for explicit lobe alignment was presented in Chapter 5. In a first step, a lobe segmentation method using level sets was proposed, in which a novel shape-based force term was introduced to attract the contour in direction of the interlobular fissures. Then, this segmentation was integrated in the basic registration framework to explicitly enforce an alignment of the lobes. In this way, shape and intensity information are combined with each other.

Using the presented segmentation-based approach, a significant improvement of lung and lobe alignment was shown for inter-subject registration based on a set of 3D CT scans. The extent of the improvement primarily depends on the quality of the lobe segmentation. For example, due to better visibility of the left fissure, segmentation was mostly superior for the left than for the right lobes. Accordingly, a more distinctive improvement of the lobe alignment was recorded for the left lung.

Varying results were obtained for intra-subject registration based on low-dose data, because the much poorer image quality impaired fissure detection and consequently lobe alignment.

Sliding motion at lung boundaries   The breathing motion causes various organs in the thorax to slide along their surrounding tissue, in particular the lung. This physiological property causes discontinuities in the transformation and therefore contradicts the employment of a homogeneous regularization scheme for the registration of thoracic CT images. Usually, this problem is implicitly addressed by restraining the registration to the lung, however, no valid transformation is provided for the background in this case. Therefore, a novel direction-dependent regularization (DDR) approach was presented in Chapter 6 to consider lung physiology by explicitly modeling sliding motion. By decoupling normal- and tangential-directed motion, discontinuities are preserved at the boundary while gaps and foldings are avoided. In the basic approach, lung boundaries are localized based on a provided segmentation. Additionally, an extension was presented to automatically detect regions in which sliding motion occurs. Finally, to circumvent the well-known drawbacks of explicit solution schemes, Fast Explicit Diffusion (FED) was adapted for solving DDR.

Registration with direction-dependent regularization was evaluated for motion estimation using various 4D CT data sets. In all cases, a significant improvement over the conventional algorithm was shown with respect to landmark alignment. The obtained accuracy was in the order of the masked registration approach but a valid transformation is provided for the whole image domain. Both DDR variants – the segmentation- and the detection-based one – performed comparably well. Furthermore, the employment of FED was shown to drastically increase accuracy and to speed up convergence.

The consideration of sliding motion between the individual lobes is principally possible with the presented methods but requires some further adjustments. In particular, artifacts arise at triple junctures where the lobes meet the lung boundaries.

Conclusion   In summary, it has been shown that the registration of thoracic CT images greatly benefits from specifically considering aspects of lung morphology and physiology. In particular, segmentations of the structures of interest provide information that can be used to either assist its alignment, or to model its physiological motion properties.

8.2 Perspectives

The methods developed in the context of this work provide several links to subsequent research projects. Some ideas are summarized in the following.

8.2.1 Optimization of the underlying registration algorithm

Several approaches can be followed to improve the basic registration algorithm that was employed throughout this thesis. Inspired by recent advances in registration, three main ideas are identified.

Modeling of further physiological properties Apart from the problems tackled in this thesis, several other possibilities exist to model characteristics of lung physiology. Current publications in this direction include for example [Gorbunova et al. 2012], where a mass-preserving distance measure is presented to account for the intensity changes caused by tissue compression. With the same purpose, Castillo et al. [2012] employ a Least Median of Squares Filtering.
A different aspect is highlighted by [Castillo et al. 2010a]. Here, the continuity of the respiratory motion is exploited by regarding the whole 4D data set instead of only image pairs to improve the registration.

Employment of advanced solution strategies Recent developments suggest that the solution strategy followed in this work bears potential for optimization. For example, discrete approaches have been successfully employed and suggest improvements to efficiency and accuracy [Cao et al. 2010b; Heinrich et al. 2012; Rühaak et al. 2013]. Moreover, they enable an intrinsic modeling of hard constraints to the transformation [Olesch et al. 2009]. Other methods aim at simultaneously solving the registration on multiple resolution levels instead of pursuing a sequential strategy as done in this work [Shi et al. 2012; Seiler et al. 2012].

Application of an automatic quality assessment A further idea to enhance registration algorithms is to employ an on-line quality assessment. This could be used to improve robustness by pointing out questionable results or to automatically select best-suited results. Some research has already been done in this direction. For example, in [Schmidt-Richberg et al. 2011] accuracy is quantified by automatically detected landmarks to optimize the regularization parameter. Muenzing et al. [2012a] use a supervised learning of local alignment patterns to assess regional registration quality. This information is then used in [Muenzing et al. 2012b] to combine registration results of different algorithms to an optimized estimate. Datteri and Dawant [2012] follow a different idea. Here, after pair-wise registration with a set of images, registration circuits are exploited to estimate the Target Registration Error (TRE).

8.2.2 Improvement of pulmonary fissure alignment

The registration approach with integrated fissure alignment presented in Chapter 5 turned out to be sensitive to the quality of the lobe segmentation, which essentially depends on the image quality and initialization. Therefore, most ideas for an improvement of the algorithm aim in that direction.

Optimization of fissure detection While fissure detection is mostly robust for normal-dose images, it remains a problem for low-dose and 4D data. Consequently, an improved fissure alignment was only obtained in part for the regarded 4D scans. Several ideas could be followed to enhance the quality of detection. For example, anatomical knowledge about the normal position of the fissures could be incorporated using a normative lung atlas [Li et al. 2012]. The consideration of regions larger than a 3×3 neighborhood for feature computation in the learning-based detection approach is also promising. Moreover, the various parameters of the classifier could be optimized to the specific data pool, which was not done in the context of this work.

Initialization based on multi-atlas segmentation Besides fissure detection, the initial level set has a major impact on the segmentation outcome. Initialization could be considerably improved using a more sophisticated atlas-based approach, as done for example in [van Rikxoort et al. 2009]. Recent advances in multi-atlas segmentation based on manifold learning promise further improvements [Wolz et al. 2010].

Consideration of vascular information The lobes are known to divide the vessel tree into separate sub-trees. Therefore, few vessels are in the proximity of the fissures [Aziz et al. 2004]. This information could be exploited by considering the vasculature in the segmentation approach, either by guiding the initialization [van Rikxoort et al. 2010] or by adding a new vessel-driven force term directly in the level set framework.

Transfer to other problems Finally, the idea of integrating segmentation information into registration algorithms using the presented joint variational framework could be applied to several other applications. In [Schmidt-Richberg et al. 2009c], it has already been successfully applied to liver registration based on CT data. Other applications include, for example, the registration of 4D heart MR images, which are very prone to noise and therefore difficult to register.

8.2.3 Extensions of sliding motion modeling

The direction-dependent regularization also has potential for optimization and application to further problems.

Lobe sliding   It would be of interest to determine the actual amount of lobe sliding in clinical 4D images representing the normal breathing cycle. In case it is of relevance, direction-dependent regularization could principally be used to assess the sliding motion. However, a handling of the artifacts described in Section 7.5 would be required.

Transfer to other problems   Moreover, the occurrence of sliding motion is evident for several other organs. In [Schmidt-Richberg et al. 2010b], direction-dependent regularization has already been successfully applied to assess liver motion. Moreover, Vandemeulebroucke et al. [2012] use motion masks of the mediastinum and organs below the diaphragm to obtain sliding motion. However, for simultaneously considering multiple structures with DDR, the aforementioned artifacts arising at triple junctures are hindering – a problem that should be tackled in future research.

Combination of fissure alignment and direction-dependent regularization
It would be interesting to combine the presented approaches for lobe alignment and direction-dependent regularization. However, a more robust segmentation would be required to obtain reliable results. In this context, it is of particular interest if an automatic detection of sliding motion between the lobes can be used to steer the segmentation algorithm.

Appendix A

On digital images

An extensive definition of digital images including the discretization problem and the interpolation of image points can be found in [Modersitzki 2004]. In this section, the focus is to establish the notations of images required for the understanding of this work.

Let a d-dimensional image be a mapping I that assigns a greyvalue to each point $\boldsymbol{x}$ of a given domain $\Omega \subset \mathbb{R}^d$:

$$I : \Omega \to \mathbb{R} \,.$$

Such a continuous representation of an image allows the definition of derivations of the image, for example the image gradient. In the clinical practice however – as in conventional photography – discretized versions of images are dealt with. Therefore, the term of a *digital image* is established. For this, the continuous image domain

$$\Omega := \,]0, N_1 h_1[\, \times \cdots \times \,]0, N_d h_d[\, \subset \mathbb{R}^d$$

with boundary $\partial\Omega$ is divided in $N = N_1 \cdots N_d$ discrete grid points $\boldsymbol{x}_{j_1,\dots,j_d} = (x_{j_1}, \dots, x_{j_d})^T$ with $1 \leq j_l \leq N_l$ and $1 \leq l \leq d$. Here, $N_l \in \mathbb{N}$ denotes the resolution and $h_l \in \mathbb{R}$ the spacing – that means the physical distance between two subsequent grid points – in direction the l-th coordinate axis. In this work, the Neumann grid is assumed, which is given by

$$\boldsymbol{x}_{j_1,\dots,j_d} := ((j_1 - 0.5)h_1, \dots, (j_d - 0.5)h_d)^T \,.$$

For various calculations it is often convenient to arrange the grid points in a vector. To this end, a lexicographical order is defined, that means a bijective mapping sending a tuple $(j_1, \dots, j_d)$ to an index j. Using a right-handed coordinate system, the most obvious choice is

$$j = j_1 + \sum_{l=2}^{d} (j_l - 1) \prod_{m=1}^{l-1} N_m \,,$$

which allows to write $\boldsymbol{x}_j = (x_{j_1}, \dots, x_{j_d})^T$. The set $\Omega^\# := \{\boldsymbol{x}_j, \ j = 1, \dots, N\} \subset \Omega$ is called the *grid*. Based on this, each grid point can be assigned to a unique corresponding point in the continuous image domain. The image value at the grid points results from a discretization process, which in this work is given by the *midpoint*

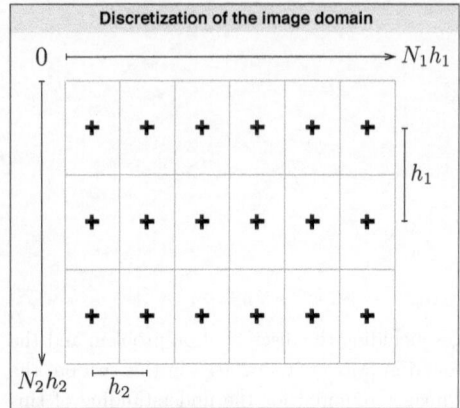
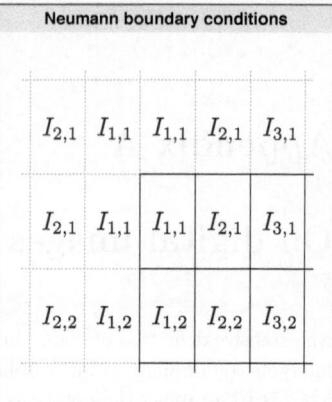

Figure A.1: Left: Illustration of the midpoint discretization with crosses indicating the discrete grid points. The image resolution in direction of the l-th coordinate axis is denoted by N_l and the corresponding spacing by h_l. Right: Illustration of Neumann boundary conditions for mid point discretization.

discretization

$$I_{j_1,\dots,j_d} = I_j := \frac{1}{|\omega(\boldsymbol{x}_j)|} \int_{\omega(\boldsymbol{x}_j)} I(\boldsymbol{x})\,d\boldsymbol{x}\,,$$

with $\omega(\boldsymbol{x}_j)$ describing a small region with the area $|\omega(\boldsymbol{x}_j)|$ and center point $\boldsymbol{x}_j$. A *digital image* $\boldsymbol{I}$ is now defined as the matrix

$$\boldsymbol{I} := (I_{j_1,\dots,j_d})_{1 \le j_l \le N_l;\ l=1,\dots,d} \in \mathbb{R}^{N_1 \times \cdots \times N_d}$$

and

$$\vec{I} := (I_j)_{j=1,\dots,N} \in \mathbb{R}^{N \times 1}$$

is called the linearized *image vector*.

To handle the boundary of the images, Neumann boundary conditions are used in this work if not stated otherwise. In the continuous domain, these can be expressed by

$$\frac{\partial I}{\partial \boldsymbol{n}}(\boldsymbol{x}) = 0 \text{ for all } \boldsymbol{x} \in \partial\Omega\,,$$

where $\boldsymbol{n}$ denotes the normal on the boundary. For the discrete setting, Neumann boundary conditions with midpoint discretization are illustrated in figure A.1. They are also called *mirroring boundary conditions*.

Appendix B

Mathematical derivations

In this appendix, some mathematical derivations are detailed concerning the calculus of variations (Appendix B.1) and the derivation of the direction-dependent regularization (Appendices B.2).

B.1 Calculus of variations

In the following section, the derivation of the Euler-Lagrange equations (ELE) required throughout this work is detailed. After a general introduction to the calculus of variations in Section B.1.1, specific terms for registration (Section B.1.2), segmentation (Section B.1.3) and the integrated framework (Section B.1.4) are regarded.

B.1.1 Derivation of the Euler-Lagrange equation

For the derivation of the Euler-Lagrange equation, first the one-dimensional case of the registration problem (3.2) with $u : \mathbb{R} \to \mathbb{R}$ is regarded. It can be reformulated to

$$\mathcal{J}[u] = \int_a^b J(u(x), u'(x), x) \, dx \tag{B.1}$$

with the boundary conditions

$$u(a) = \alpha \quad \text{und} \quad u(b) = \beta \, .$$

The dependence of u on x is omitted in the following to enhance readability. A minimum of the functional is reached, if the variations of u in all directions v with $v(a) = v(b) = 0$ are zero, that means

$$0 = \delta \mathcal{J}[u; v] = \frac{d}{d\epsilon} \mathcal{J}[u + \epsilon v] \Big|_{\epsilon=0}$$
$$= \int_a^b \frac{\partial}{\partial \epsilon} J(u + \epsilon v, u' + \epsilon v', x) \Big|_{\epsilon=0} dx$$

$$= \int_a^b \lim_{\epsilon \to 0} \frac{1}{\epsilon} \left(J(u + \epsilon v, u' + \epsilon v', x) - J(u, u', x) \right) dx$$

$$= \int_a^b \left(J(u, u', x) + \frac{\partial J}{\partial u} v + \frac{\partial J}{\partial u'} v' - J(u, u', x) \right) dx$$

$$= \int_a^b \left(\frac{\partial J}{\partial u} v + \frac{\partial J}{\partial u'} v' \right) dx \,.$$

The second summand in the last row can be reformulated by integration by parts to

$$\int_a^b \frac{\partial J}{\partial u'} v' \, dx = \left[\frac{\partial J}{\partial u'} v \right]_a^b - \int_a^b \frac{d}{dx} \left(\frac{\partial J}{\partial u'} \right) v \, dx = - \int_a^b \frac{d}{dx} \left(\frac{\partial J}{\partial u'} \right) v \, dx \,,$$

which leads to

$$0 = \delta \mathcal{J}[u; v] = \int_a^b \left(\frac{\partial J}{\partial u} - \frac{d}{dx} \frac{\partial J}{\partial u'} \right) v \, dx \,. \tag{B.2}$$

Since equation (B.2) has to hold for all v, the integrand has to equal zero. A condition for a minimum of (B.1) is therefore

$$0 = \frac{\partial J}{\partial u} - \frac{d}{dx} \frac{\partial J}{\partial u'} \,. \tag{B.3}$$

This is called the *first-order Euler-Lagrange equation*.

B.1.1.1 Multi-dimensional functions

To obtain a generalization of the Euler-Lagrange equation, multi-dimensional functions $\boldsymbol{u} : \mathbb{R} \to \mathbb{R}^d$ with $\boldsymbol{u}(x) = (u_1(x), \dots, u_d(x))^T$ are considered in the next step. The energy functional then reads

$$\mathcal{J}[\boldsymbol{u}] = \int_a^b J(\boldsymbol{u}, u_1', \dots, u_d', x) \, dx \,.$$

Here, the neighboring functions $u_l(x) + \epsilon v_l(x)$ have to be considered for all $l = 1, \dots, d$ components. The corresponding condition then reads

$$0 = \delta \mathcal{J}[\boldsymbol{u}; \boldsymbol{v}] = \int_a^b \frac{\partial}{\partial \epsilon} J(u_1 + \epsilon v_1, \dots, u_d + \epsilon v_d, u_1' + \epsilon v_1', \dots, u_d' + \epsilon v_d', x) \Big|_{\epsilon = 0} dx \,,$$

which leads to the Euler-Lagrange equations

$$0 = \frac{\partial J}{\partial u_l} - \frac{d}{dx} \frac{\partial J}{\partial u_l'} \qquad l = 1, \dots, d$$

for all l components.

B.1.1.2 Functions of several variables

In the last step, functions of several variables $\boldsymbol{u} : \mathbb{R}^d \to \mathbb{R}^d$ are considered. Equation (B.1) then reads

$$\mathcal{J}[\boldsymbol{u}] = \int_\Omega J(\boldsymbol{u}, \nabla u_1, \ldots, \nabla u_d, \boldsymbol{x}) \, d\boldsymbol{x}$$

and it is

$$0 = \delta \mathcal{J}[\boldsymbol{u}; \boldsymbol{v}] = \int_\Omega \left(\frac{\partial J}{\partial u_l} v_l + \sum_{i=1}^d \frac{\partial J}{\partial(\partial_{x_i} u_l)} \frac{\partial v_l}{\partial x_i} \right) d\boldsymbol{x} \qquad l = 1, \ldots, d,$$

with $\partial_{x_i} v_l := \frac{\partial v_l}{\partial x_i}$. Applying integration by parts to the second term of the integrand gives the convergence theorem

$$\int_\Omega \frac{\partial J}{\partial(\partial_{x_i} u_l)} \frac{\partial v_l}{\partial x_i} \, d\boldsymbol{x} = \int_{\partial\Omega} \frac{\partial J}{\partial(\partial_{x_i} u_l)} v_l \, n_i \, d\boldsymbol{x} - \int_\Omega \frac{\partial}{\partial x_i} \frac{\partial J}{\partial(\partial_{x_i} u_l)} \, v_l \, d\boldsymbol{x},$$

where n_i is the ith component of the outwards directed normal vector $\boldsymbol{n}$. The imposed boundary condition $\boldsymbol{v} = 0$ on $\partial\Omega$ finally leads to

$$0 = \frac{\partial J}{\partial u_l} - \sum_{i=1}^d \frac{\partial}{\partial x_i} \frac{\partial J}{\partial(\partial_{x_i} u_l)} \qquad l = 1, \ldots, d. \tag{B.4}$$

This is the Euler-Lagrange equation in generalized form. If no boundary conditions are explicitly imposed, the second term only disappears if the *natural boundary conditions*

$$0 = \int_{\partial\Omega} \left\langle \frac{\partial J}{\partial(\partial_{\boldsymbol{x}} u_l)}, \boldsymbol{n} \right\rangle d\boldsymbol{x} \qquad l = 1, \ldots, d$$

hold.

B.1.2 Derivation of registration terms

B.1.2.1 Sum of Squared Differences

The SSD distance measure (3.11)

$$\mathcal{D}[R, T; \boldsymbol{u}] = \frac{1}{2} \int_\Omega (R(\boldsymbol{x}) - T(\boldsymbol{x} - \boldsymbol{u}(\boldsymbol{x})))^2 \, d\boldsymbol{x}$$

does not depend on derivatives of the displacement $\boldsymbol{u}$. The Euler-Lagrange equation (B.4) therefore simplifies to

$$0 = \frac{\partial D}{\partial u_l} \qquad l = 1, \ldots, d$$

with $\mathcal{D}[R, T; \boldsymbol{u}] = \int_\Omega D[\boldsymbol{u}] \, d\boldsymbol{x}$. It is

$$\frac{\partial D}{\partial u_l} = \frac{\partial}{\partial u_l} \frac{1}{2} (R(\boldsymbol{x}) - T(\boldsymbol{x} - \boldsymbol{u}(\boldsymbol{x})))^2$$

$$= (R(\boldsymbol{x}) - T(\boldsymbol{x} - \boldsymbol{u}(\boldsymbol{x}))) \frac{\partial}{\partial u_l} (R(\boldsymbol{x}) - T(\boldsymbol{x} - \boldsymbol{u}(\boldsymbol{x})))$$

$$= -(R(\boldsymbol{x}) - T(\boldsymbol{x} - \boldsymbol{u}(\boldsymbol{x}))) \nabla T(\boldsymbol{x} - \boldsymbol{u}(\boldsymbol{x})) \cdot \frac{\partial}{\partial u_l} (\boldsymbol{x} - \boldsymbol{u}(\boldsymbol{x}))$$

$$= (R(\boldsymbol{x}) - T(\boldsymbol{x} - \boldsymbol{u}(\boldsymbol{x}))) \nabla T(\boldsymbol{x} - \boldsymbol{u}(\boldsymbol{x})) \cdot \boldsymbol{e}_l \,,$$

with $\boldsymbol{e}_l$ denoting the l-th unity vector. This can be abbreviated to

$$\boldsymbol{f}^{SSD} = (D_{u_1}, \dots, D_{u_d})^T = (R(\boldsymbol{x}) - T(\boldsymbol{x} - \boldsymbol{u}(\boldsymbol{x}))) \nabla T(\boldsymbol{x} - \boldsymbol{u}(\boldsymbol{x})) \,.$$

B.1.2.2 Diffusion regularization

The diffusion regularization (3.15) is given by $\mathcal{S}[\boldsymbol{u}] = \int_\Omega S[\boldsymbol{u}] \, d\boldsymbol{x}$ with

$$S[\boldsymbol{u}] = \frac{1}{2} \sum_{k=1}^d \|\nabla u_k\|^2 = \frac{1}{2} \sum_{k=1}^d \sum_{j=1}^d \left(\frac{\partial}{\partial x_j} u_k \right)^2 \,.$$

Since this term only depends on the derivatives of $\boldsymbol{u}$, the Euler-Lagrange equation simplifies to

$$0 = -\sum_{i=1}^d \frac{\partial}{\partial x_i} \frac{\partial S}{\partial (\partial_{x_i} u_l)} \qquad l = 1, \dots, d$$

It is

$$-\sum_{i=1}^d \frac{\partial}{\partial x_i} \frac{\partial S}{\partial (\partial_{x_i} u_l)} = -\sum_{i=1}^d \frac{\partial}{\partial x_i} \left(\frac{\partial}{\partial (\frac{\partial}{\partial x_i} u_l)} \frac{1}{2} \sum_{k=1}^d \sum_{j=1}^d \left(\frac{\partial}{\partial x_j} u_k \right)^2 \right)$$

$$= -\sum_{i=1}^d \frac{\partial}{\partial x_i} \left(\frac{\partial}{\partial (\frac{\partial}{\partial x_i} u_l)} \frac{1}{2} \sum_{j=1}^d \left(\frac{\partial}{\partial x_j} u_l \right)^2 \right)$$

$$= -\sum_{i=1}^d \frac{\partial}{\partial x_i} \left(\frac{\partial}{\partial (\frac{\partial}{\partial x_i} u_l)} \frac{1}{2} \left(\frac{\partial}{\partial x_i} u_l \right)^2 \right)$$

$$= -\sum_{i=1}^d \frac{\partial}{\partial x_i} \frac{\partial}{\partial x_i} u_l$$

$$= -\Delta u_l$$

for all l, leading to

$$\nabla \mathcal{S}^{diff}[\boldsymbol{u}] = \mathcal{A}^{diff} \boldsymbol{u} = \Delta \boldsymbol{u} \,,$$

with $\Delta \boldsymbol{u} := (\Delta u_1, \dots, \Delta u_d)^T$.

B.1.2.3 Anisotropic diffusion regularization

Before regarding the direction-dependent regularization, anisotropic diffusion is derived [Weickert et al. 1998]. Here, the amount of smoothing is weighted with a spatially varying function $\omega : \Omega \to [0, 1]$. The regularizer then reads

$$S^\omega[\boldsymbol{u}] = \frac{1}{2} \sum_{k=1}^{d} \omega \left\| \nabla u_k \right\|^2 = \frac{1}{2} \sum_{k=1}^{d} \omega \sum_{j=1}^{d} \left(\frac{\partial}{\partial x_j} u_k \right)^2 .$$

Equivalently to the diffusion registration, deriving the Euler-Lagrange equation leads to

$$-\sum_{i=1}^{d} \frac{\partial}{\partial x_i} \frac{\partial S^\omega}{\partial(\partial_{x_i} u_l)} = -\sum_{i=1}^{d} \frac{\partial}{\partial x_i} \omega \frac{\partial S}{\partial(\partial_{x_i} u_l)}$$

$$= -\sum_{i=1}^{d} \frac{\partial}{\partial x_i} \omega \frac{\partial}{\partial x_i} u_l$$

$$= -\nabla \cdot (\omega \nabla u_l)$$

and finally

$$\nabla S^\omega[\boldsymbol{u}] = \mathcal{A}^\omega \boldsymbol{u} = \nabla \cdot (\omega \nabla \boldsymbol{u}) ,$$

which is simplified to $\nabla \omega \nabla \boldsymbol{u}$ in the following.

B.1.2.4 Direction-dependent regularization

The direction-dependent regularization defined by (6.2) and (6.8) can be reformulated to

$$S^{DDR}[\boldsymbol{u}] = \int_\Omega \omega S^\perp[\boldsymbol{u}] + (1 - \omega) S[\boldsymbol{u}] \, d\boldsymbol{x} + \sum_i \int_{\Gamma_i} \omega S^\parallel[\boldsymbol{u}] \, d\boldsymbol{x} .$$

To begin with, $S^\perp$ and $S^\parallel$ are regarded separately. It is

$$S^\perp[\boldsymbol{u}] = \frac{1}{2} \sum_{k=1}^{d} \left\| \nabla \langle \boldsymbol{u}, \boldsymbol{n} \rangle n_k \right\|^2$$

$$= \frac{1}{2} \sum_{k=1}^{d} \sum_{j=1}^{d} \left(\frac{\partial}{\partial x_j} \sum_{m=1}^{d} u_m n_m n_k \right)^2 .$$

If $\boldsymbol{n}$ is assumed to be independent of $\boldsymbol{x}$,

$$\left(\frac{\partial}{\partial x_j} \sum_{m=1}^{d} u_m n_m n_k \right)^2 = n_k^2 \left(\frac{\partial}{\partial x_j} \sum_{m=1}^{d} u_m n_m \right)^2$$

is valid. Exploiting $\sum_k n_k^2 = 1$, the system of Euler-Lagrange equations for $l = 1, \ldots, d$ is derived by:

$$
\begin{aligned}
-\sum_{i=1}^{d} \frac{\partial}{\partial x_i} \frac{\partial S^{\perp}}{\partial(\partial_{x_i} u_l)} &= -\sum_{i=1}^{d} \frac{\partial}{\partial x_i} \left(\frac{\partial}{\partial(\frac{\partial}{\partial x_i} u_l)} \frac{1}{2} \sum_{k=1}^{d} \sum_{j=1}^{d} n_k^2 \left(\sum_{m=1}^{d} \frac{\partial}{\partial x_j} u_m n_m \right)^2 \right) \\
&= -\sum_{i=1}^{d} \frac{\partial}{\partial x_i} \left(\frac{\partial}{\partial(\frac{\partial}{\partial x_i} u_l)} \frac{1}{2} \sum_{j=1}^{d} \left(\sum_{m=1}^{d} \frac{\partial}{\partial x_j} u_m n_m \right)^2 \right) \\
&= -\sum_{i=1}^{d} \frac{\partial}{\partial x_i} \left(\frac{\partial}{\partial(\frac{\partial}{\partial x_i} u_l)} \frac{1}{2} \left(\sum_{m=1}^{d} \frac{\partial}{\partial x_i} u_m n_m \right)^2 \right) \\
&= -\sum_{i=1}^{d} \frac{\partial}{\partial x_i} \left(\sum_{m=1}^{d} \frac{\partial}{\partial x_i} u_m n_m \right) n_l \\
&= -\sum_{i=1}^{d} \frac{\partial}{\partial x_i} \frac{\partial}{\partial x_i} \left(\sum_{m=1}^{d} u_m n_m \right) n_l \\
&= -\Delta \langle \boldsymbol{u}, \boldsymbol{n} \rangle n_l
\end{aligned}
$$

and

$$
\mathcal{A}^{\perp} \boldsymbol{u}^{\perp} = \mathcal{A}^{diff} \boldsymbol{u}^{\perp} = \Delta \boldsymbol{u}^{\perp}.
$$

Equivalently, $S^{\parallel}$ can be written as

$$
\begin{aligned}
S^{\parallel}[\boldsymbol{u}] &= \frac{1}{2} \sum_{k=1}^{d} \| \nabla \left(u_k - \langle \boldsymbol{u}, \boldsymbol{n} \rangle n_k \right) \|^2 \\
&= \frac{1}{2} \sum_{k=1}^{d} \sum_{j=1}^{d} \left[\frac{\partial}{\partial x_j} \left(u_k - \sum_{m=1}^{d} u_m n_m n_k \right) \right]^2.
\end{aligned}
$$

For deriving the corresponding Euler-Lagrange equation, the second part is first considered separately:

$$
\begin{aligned}
\frac{\partial S^{\parallel}}{\partial(\partial_{x_i} u_l)} &= \frac{\partial}{\partial(\frac{\partial}{\partial x_i} u_l)} \frac{1}{2} \sum_{k=1}^{d} \sum_{j=1}^{d} \left(\frac{\partial}{\partial x_j} u_k - \frac{\partial}{\partial x_j} \langle \boldsymbol{u}, \boldsymbol{n} \rangle n_k \right)^2 \\
&= \frac{\partial}{\partial(\frac{\partial}{\partial x_i} u_l)} \frac{1}{2} \sum_{k=1}^{d} \left(\frac{\partial}{\partial x_i} u_k - \frac{\partial}{\partial x_i} \langle \boldsymbol{u}, \boldsymbol{n} \rangle n_k \right)^2 \\
&= \frac{\partial}{\partial(\frac{\partial}{\partial x_i} u_l)} \left[\frac{1}{2} \sum_{k=1}^{d} \left(\frac{\partial}{\partial x_i} u_k \right)^2 + \frac{1}{2} \sum_{k=1}^{d} n_k^2 \left(\frac{\partial}{\partial x_i} \langle \boldsymbol{u}, \boldsymbol{n} \rangle \right)^2 \right. \\
&\qquad \left. - \sum_{k=1}^{d} \left(\frac{\partial}{\partial x_i} u_k \right) \left(\frac{\partial}{\partial x_i} \langle \boldsymbol{u}, \boldsymbol{n} \rangle n_k \right) \right] \\
&= \frac{\partial}{\partial(\frac{\partial}{\partial x_i} u_l)} \left[\frac{1}{2} \left(\frac{\partial}{\partial x_i} u_l \right)^2 + \frac{1}{2} \left(\frac{\partial}{\partial x_i} \langle \boldsymbol{u}, \boldsymbol{n} \rangle \right)^2 \right.
\end{aligned}
$$

$$-\sum_{k=1}^{d}\left(\frac{\partial}{\partial x_i}u_k\right)\left(\frac{\partial}{\partial x_i}\langle \boldsymbol{u}, \boldsymbol{n}\rangle n_k\right)\Big]$$

$$=\left(\frac{\partial}{\partial x_i}u_l\right)+n_l\left(\frac{\partial}{\partial x_i}\langle \boldsymbol{u}, \boldsymbol{n}\rangle\right)-2n_l\left(\frac{\partial}{\partial x_i}\langle \boldsymbol{u}, \boldsymbol{n}\rangle\right)$$

$$=\frac{\partial}{\partial x_i}\left(u_l-\langle \boldsymbol{u}, \boldsymbol{n}\rangle n_l\right),$$

whereat the product rule $(ab)' = a'b + ab'$ is applied to write

$$\frac{\partial}{\partial(\frac{\partial}{\partial x_i}u_l)}\sum_{k=1}^{d}\left(\frac{\partial}{\partial x_i}u_k\right)\left(\frac{\partial}{\partial x_i}\sum_{m=1}^{d}u_m n_m n_k\right)=\frac{\partial}{\partial x_i}\langle \boldsymbol{u}, \boldsymbol{n}\rangle\,n_l+\sum_{k=1}^{d}\left(\frac{\partial}{\partial x_i}u_k\right)n_l n_k$$

$$=\frac{\partial}{\partial x_i}\langle \boldsymbol{u}, \boldsymbol{n}\rangle\,n_l+n_l\frac{\partial}{\partial x_i}\langle \boldsymbol{u}, \boldsymbol{n}\rangle$$

$$=2n_l\frac{\partial}{\partial x_i}\langle \boldsymbol{u}, \boldsymbol{n}\rangle\,.$$

Inserting this in the Euler-Lagrange equation gives

$$-\sum_{i=1}^{d}\frac{\partial}{\partial x_i}\frac{\partial S^{\|}}{\partial(\partial_{x_i}u_l)}=-\sum_{i=1}^{d}\frac{\partial}{\partial x_i}\frac{\partial}{\partial x_i}\left(u_l-\langle \boldsymbol{u}, \boldsymbol{n}\rangle n_l\right)$$

$$=-\Delta(u_l-\langle \boldsymbol{u}, \boldsymbol{n}\rangle n_l)$$

and finally

$$\mathcal{A}^{\|}\boldsymbol{u}^{\|}=\mathcal{A}^{diff}\boldsymbol{u}^{\|}=\Delta\boldsymbol{u}^{\|}\,.$$

Next, the weighting function ω is included in analogy to Section B.1.2.3. This yields $\mathcal{A}^{\|,\omega}\boldsymbol{u}^{\|}=\nabla\omega\nabla\boldsymbol{u}^{\|}$ and $\mathcal{A}^{\perp,\omega}\boldsymbol{u}^{\perp}=\nabla\omega\nabla\boldsymbol{u}^{\perp}$, and accordingly

$$\nabla\mathcal{S}^{DDR}[\boldsymbol{u}]=\mathcal{A}^{DDR}[\boldsymbol{u}]=\nabla\omega\nabla\boldsymbol{u}^{\perp}\;+\;\nabla(1-\omega)\nabla\boldsymbol{u}\;+\;\widehat{\nabla}\omega\widehat{\nabla}\boldsymbol{u}^{\|}\,.$$

Here, to incorporate the splitting of the image domain in equation 6.2, $\widehat{\nabla}$ denotes that the gradient is computed for each object Σ_i using Neumann boundary conditions.

B.1.3 Derivation of segmentation terms

Since the level set function is not vector-valued, the Euler-Lagrange equation (B.4) simplifies to

$$0=\frac{\partial J}{\partial\phi}-\sum_{i=1}^{d}\frac{\partial}{\partial x_i}\frac{\partial J}{\partial(\partial_{x_i}\phi)}.\qquad\qquad(B.5)$$

The specific energy terms are regarded in the following.

B.1.3.1 Internal energy

The internal energy (4.3) is defined by $\mathcal{I}[\phi] = \int_\Omega I[\phi]\,d\boldsymbol{x}$ with

$$I[\phi] = \delta(\phi)\,\|\nabla\phi\|\,.$$

The derivation of the Euler-Lagrange equation (B.5) requires the computation of the terms

$$I_\phi := \frac{\partial I}{\partial \phi} = \delta'(\phi)\|\nabla\phi\|$$

and

$$\begin{aligned}
I_{\partial_{x_i}\phi} &:= \frac{\partial I}{\partial(\partial_{x_i}\phi)} \\
&= \delta(\phi)\,\frac{\partial}{\partial(\partial_{x_i}\phi)}\left(\sum_{j=1}^{d}(\partial_{x_j}\phi)^2\right)^{\frac{1}{2}} \\
&= \delta(\phi)\,\frac{\partial\phi}{\partial x_i}\frac{1}{\|\nabla\phi\|}\,,
\end{aligned}$$

whereat $\|\nabla\phi(\boldsymbol{x})\| \neq 0$ is assumed in the last equality. Substituting these terms in (B.5) yields

$$\begin{aligned}
I_\phi - \sum_{i=1}^{d}\frac{\partial}{\partial x_i}I_{\partial_{x_i}\phi} &= \delta'(\phi)\|\nabla\phi\| \; - \; \sum_{i=1}^{d}\frac{\partial}{\partial x_i}\left(\delta(\phi)\frac{\partial\phi}{\partial x_i}\frac{1}{\|\nabla\phi\|}\right) \\
&= \delta'(\phi)\|\nabla\phi\| \; - \; \sum_{i=1}^{d}\left(\frac{\partial\phi}{\partial x_i}\frac{1}{\|\nabla\phi\|}\frac{\partial}{\partial x_i}\delta(\phi) \; + \; \delta(\phi)\frac{\partial}{\partial x_i}\left(\frac{\partial\phi}{\partial x_i}\frac{1}{\|\nabla\phi\|}\right)\right) \\
&= \delta'(\phi)\|\nabla\phi\| \; - \; \sum_{i=1}^{d}\left(\delta'(\phi)\left(\frac{\partial\phi}{\partial x_i}\right)^2\frac{1}{\|\nabla\phi\|} \; + \; \delta(\phi)\frac{\partial}{\partial x_i}\frac{\frac{\partial}{\partial x_i}\phi}{\|\nabla\phi\|}\right) \\
&= \delta'(\phi)\|\nabla\phi\| \; - \; \delta'(\phi)\frac{\sum_{i=1}^{d}\left(\frac{\partial\phi}{\partial x_i}\right)^2}{\|\nabla\phi\|} \; - \; \delta(\phi)\sum_{i=1}^{d}\frac{\partial}{\partial x_i}\frac{\frac{\partial}{\partial x_i}\phi}{\|\nabla\phi\|} \\
&= \delta'(\phi)\|\nabla\phi\| \; - \; \delta'(\phi)\frac{\|\nabla\phi\|^2}{\|\nabla\phi\|} \; - \; \delta(\phi)\nabla\cdot\frac{\nabla\phi}{\|\nabla\phi\|} \\
&= -\,\delta(\phi)\nabla\cdot\frac{\nabla\phi}{\|\nabla\phi\|}\,.
\end{aligned}$$

Finally, the Euler-Lagrange equation is given by

$$0 = \nabla\mathcal{I}[\phi] = -\,\delta(\phi)\nabla\cdot\frac{\nabla\phi}{\|\nabla\phi\|}\,.$$

B.1.3.2 External energy

The external energy (4.4) is given by $\mathcal{E}[I;\phi] = \int_\Omega E[\phi]\,d\boldsymbol{x}$ with

$$E[\phi] = H(\phi) \cdot \log(p_{out}(I)) + (1 - H(\phi)) \cdot \log(p_{in}(I)).$$

Since E does not depend on derivatives of ϕ, equation (B.5) simplifies to

$$
\begin{aligned}
E_\phi := \frac{\partial E}{\partial \phi} &= \frac{\partial}{\partial \phi}\, H(\phi) \cdot \log(p_{out}(I)) \;+\; \frac{\partial}{\partial \phi}\,(1 - H(\phi)) \cdot \log(p_{in}(I)) \\
&= \delta(\phi) \cdot \log(p_{out}(I)) \;-\; \delta(\phi) \cdot \log(p_{in}(I)).
\end{aligned}
$$

The Euler-Lagrange equation is then given by

$$0 = \nabla \mathcal{E}[I;\phi] = \delta(\phi) \cdot \log(p_{out}(I)) \;-\; \delta(\phi) \cdot \log(p_{in}(I)).$$

B.1.3.3 Prior shape term

The Euler-Lagrange equation of the prior shape term $\mathcal{P}[\tilde{\phi};\phi] = \int_\Omega P[\phi]\,d\boldsymbol{x}$ with

$$P[\phi] = \frac{1}{2}\,\delta(\phi)\left(\tilde{\phi} - \phi\right)^2$$

simplifies to

$$
\begin{aligned}
P_\phi := \frac{\partial P}{\partial \phi} &= \frac{\partial}{\partial \phi}\,\frac{1}{2}\,\delta(\phi)\left(\tilde{\phi} - \phi\right)^2 \\
&= \frac{1}{2}\,\delta(\phi)\,\frac{\partial}{\partial \phi}\left(\tilde{\phi} - \phi\right)^2 + \frac{1}{2}\left(\tilde{\phi} - \phi\right)^2\,\frac{\partial}{\partial \phi}\delta(\phi) \\
&= \delta(\phi)\left(\tilde{\phi} - \phi\right) - \frac{1}{2}\left(\tilde{\phi} - \phi\right)^2\,\delta'(\phi).
\end{aligned}
$$

Accordingly, the resulting force consists of two terms. The first term $\delta(\phi)(\tilde{\phi} - \phi)$ shows the expected behavior: If $\tilde{\phi} < \phi$ – that means if the boundary of ϕ is inside the object $\tilde{\phi}$ – the update value is negative and the zero level set of ϕ propagates outwards. In the opposite case $\tilde{\phi} > \phi$, the boundary moves inwards.

The second term $-\frac{1}{2}(\tilde{\phi} - \phi)^2\,\delta'(\phi)$, however, aims at minimizing the energy by multiplication with δ' and thereby increasing the slope of ϕ around the zero level set to decrease the distance to $\tilde{\phi}$. Since this does not induce a propagation of the boundary, the term is disregarded and the Euler-Lagrange equation approximated by

$$0 = \nabla \mathcal{P}[\tilde{\phi};\phi] \approx \delta(\phi)\left(\tilde{\phi} - \phi\right).$$

B.1.3.4 Gradient term

The gradient term $\mathcal{G}[E;\phi] = \int_\Omega G[\phi]\,d\boldsymbol{x}$ introduced in Section 4.2.2 is characterized by

$$G = (H(\phi) - 0.5)\nabla\phi \cdot \nabla E = (H(\phi) - 0.5)\sum_{j=1}^{d} \frac{\partial\phi}{\partial x_j}\frac{\partial E}{\partial x_j}\,.$$

For the Euler-Lagrange equation, first the terms

$$G_\phi := \frac{\partial G}{\partial\phi} = \delta(\phi)\nabla\phi \cdot \nabla E$$

and

$$G_{\partial_{x_i}\phi} := \frac{\partial G}{\partial(\partial_{x_i}\phi)} = (H(\phi) - 0.5)\frac{\partial}{\partial(\partial_{x_i}\phi)}\sum_{j=1}^{d}\frac{\partial\phi}{\partial x_j}\frac{\partial E}{\partial x_j}$$

$$= (H(\phi) - 0.5)\frac{\partial E}{\partial x_i}$$

are derived. Substitution in (B.5) yields

$$G_\phi - \sum_{i=1}^{d}\frac{\partial}{\partial x_i}G_{\partial_{x_i}\phi} = \delta(\phi)\nabla\phi \cdot \nabla E - \sum_{i=1}^{d}\frac{\partial}{\partial x_i}(H(\phi) - 0.5)\frac{\partial E}{\partial x_i}$$

$$= \delta(\phi)\nabla\phi \cdot \nabla E - (H(\phi) - 0.5)\Delta E\,.$$

Similarly to Appendix B.1.3.3, the equation consists of two terms. The first term $\delta(\phi)\nabla\phi \cdot \nabla E$ forces the boundary in the direction of the edge, which is the intended behavior. However, $(H(\phi)-0.5)\Delta E$ induces a steepening of the slope of ϕ. In accordance with the previous section, this term is therefore disregarded and the Euler-Lagrange equation approximated by

$$0 = \nabla\mathcal{G}[E;\phi] \approx \delta(\phi)\nabla\phi \cdot \nabla E\,.$$

B.1.4 Derivation of the terms of the joint framework

For the consistency condition defined in Section 5.1.2 it is

$$P[\phi_B;\varphi,\phi_I] := \frac{1}{2}\delta(\phi_I)\left(\phi_B \circ \varphi - \phi_I\right)^2\,.$$

Since this term combines segmentation and registration, it has to be derived in direction of the level set function ϕ_I and the displacement field $\boldsymbol{u}$, that means

$$P_{\phi_I} := \frac{\partial P}{\partial\phi_I} \quad\text{and}\quad P_{u_l} := \frac{\partial P}{\partial u_l}$$

are sought. In accordance to the prior shape term in Section B.1.3.3, it is

$$P_{\phi_I} = \delta(\phi)\,(\phi_B \circ \varphi - \phi_I)\;-\frac{1}{2}\,(\phi_B \circ \varphi - \phi_I)^2\;\delta'(\phi_I)$$

and thus

$$0 = \nabla_{\phi_I}\mathcal{P}[\phi_B;\varphi,\phi_I] \approx \delta(\phi)\,(\phi_B \circ \varphi - \phi_I)\;.$$

For the registration component, it is

$$\begin{aligned}
P_{u_l} &= \frac{\partial}{\partial u_l}\frac{1}{2}\delta(\phi_I(\boldsymbol{x}))\,\Big(\phi_B(\boldsymbol{x}-\boldsymbol{u}(\boldsymbol{x}))-\phi_I(\boldsymbol{x})\Big)^2\\
&= \frac{1}{2}\delta(\phi_I(\boldsymbol{x}))\,\frac{\partial}{\partial u_l}\Big(\phi_B(\boldsymbol{x}-\boldsymbol{u}(\boldsymbol{x}))-\phi_I(\boldsymbol{x})\Big)^2\\
&= \delta(\phi_I(\boldsymbol{x}))\,\Big(\phi_I(\boldsymbol{x})-\phi_B(\boldsymbol{x}-\boldsymbol{u}(\boldsymbol{x}))\Big)\,\nabla\phi_B(\boldsymbol{x}-\boldsymbol{u}(\boldsymbol{x}))\cdot\boldsymbol{e}_l\;,
\end{aligned}$$

which leads to

$$0 = \nabla_{\boldsymbol{u}}\mathcal{P}[\phi_B;\varphi,\phi_I] = \delta(\phi_I)\,\Big(\phi_I-\phi_B\circ\varphi\Big)\,\nabla(\phi_B\circ\varphi).$$

B.2 Derivation of DDR

In the following, the reformulation (6.1) of the diffusion regularization is detailed. It is

$$\begin{aligned}
\|\nabla u_l\|^2 &= \sum_{k=1}^d\left(\frac{\partial}{\partial x_k}u_l\right)^2\\
&= \sum_{k=1}^d\left(\frac{\partial}{\partial x_k}(u_l-\langle\boldsymbol{u},\boldsymbol{n}\rangle\,n_l+\langle\boldsymbol{u},\boldsymbol{n}\rangle\,n_l)\right)^2\\
&= \sum_{k=1}^d\left(\left(\frac{\partial}{\partial x_k}(u_l-\langle\boldsymbol{u},\boldsymbol{n}\rangle\,n_l)\right)^2+\left(\frac{\partial}{\partial x_k}\langle\boldsymbol{u},\boldsymbol{n}\rangle\,n_l\right)^2\right.\\
&\qquad\left.+2\left(\frac{\partial}{\partial x_k}(u_l-\langle\boldsymbol{u},\boldsymbol{n}\rangle\,n_l)\right)\left(\frac{\partial}{\partial x_k}\langle\boldsymbol{u},\boldsymbol{n}\rangle\,n_l\right)\right)\\
&= \|\nabla u_l^\parallel\|^2+\|\nabla u_l^\perp\|^2+2\left\langle\nabla u_l^\parallel,\nabla u_l^\perp\right\rangle
\end{aligned}$$

For the diffusion regularization, this leads to

$$\begin{aligned}
\mathcal{S}^{diff}[\varphi] &= \frac{1}{2}\sum_{l=1}^d\int_\Omega\|\nabla u_l\|^2\,d\boldsymbol{x}\\
&= \frac{1}{2}\sum_{l=1}^d\int_\Omega\|\nabla u_l^\perp\|^2\;+\;\|\nabla u_l^\parallel\|^2\,d\boldsymbol{x}+\int_\Omega\sum_{l=1}^d\left\langle\nabla u_l^\parallel,\nabla u_l^\perp\right\rangle\,d\boldsymbol{x}\;.
\end{aligned}$$

Under the assumption that $\boldsymbol{n}$ is independent of $\boldsymbol{x}$, the integrand of the second term can be reformulated to

$$
\begin{aligned}
\sum_{l=1}^{d} \left\langle \nabla u_l^{\parallel}, \nabla u_l^{\perp} \right\rangle &= \sum_{l=1}^{d} \sum_{k=1}^{d} \left(\frac{\partial}{\partial x_k} (u_l - \langle \boldsymbol{u}, \boldsymbol{n} \rangle n_l) \right) \left(\frac{\partial}{\partial x_k} \langle \boldsymbol{u}, \boldsymbol{n} \rangle n_l \right) \\
&= \sum_{l=1}^{d} \sum_{k=1}^{d} \left(\frac{\partial}{\partial x_k} u_l \frac{\partial}{\partial x_k} \langle \boldsymbol{u}, \boldsymbol{n} \rangle n_l - \frac{\partial}{\partial x_k} \langle \boldsymbol{u}, \boldsymbol{n} \rangle n_l \frac{\partial}{\partial x_k} \langle \boldsymbol{u}, \boldsymbol{n} \rangle n_l \right) \\
&= \sum_{l=1}^{d} \sum_{k=1}^{d} \frac{\partial}{\partial x_k} u_l n_l \frac{\partial}{\partial x_k} \langle \boldsymbol{u}, \boldsymbol{n} \rangle - \sum_{l=1}^{d} n_l^2 \sum_{k=1}^{d} \left(\frac{\partial}{\partial x_k} \langle \boldsymbol{u}, \boldsymbol{n} \rangle \right)^2 \\
&= \sum_{k=1}^{d} \left(\frac{\partial}{\partial x_k} \langle \boldsymbol{u}, \boldsymbol{n} \rangle \right)^2 - 1 \cdot \sum_{k=1}^{d} \left(\frac{\partial}{\partial x_k} \langle \boldsymbol{u}, \boldsymbol{n} \rangle \right)^2 = 0
\end{aligned}
$$

Consequently, the equation (6.1) is true under the given assumption.

Appendix C

Supplementary results

Table C.1: Detailed results of the LAE for the DIR-lab data in Table 7.1. All results were generated with masked active NSSD forces and diffusion regularization.

Dataset	Before registr.	Until convergence			10 Minutes runtime		
		Expl.	SI	FED	Expl.	SI	FED
Case 01	3.892	1.226	1.184	1.181	1.226	1.184	1.139
Case 02	4.338	1.136	1.102	1.097	1.136	1.102	1.135
Case 03	6.943	1.321	1.290	1.285	1.321	1.290	1.330
Case 04	9.830	2.869	1.975	2.275	2.869	1.975	3.167
Case 05	7.477	1.515	1.516	1.490	1.515	1.516	1.541
Case 06	10.89	2.385	1.705	1.877	3.662	2.938	2.039
Case 07	11.03	2.314	1.874	1.959	2.859	3.028	2.011
Case 08	14.99	1.909	1.607	1.505	2.274	2.220	1.714
Case 09	7.918	2.105	1.632	1.691	2.818	1.891	1.912
Case 10	7.301	1.534	1.437	1.394	1.734	1.942	1.472
Average	8.461	1.831	1.532	1.575	2.142	1.909	1.771

Table C.2: Detailed results of the LAE for the DIR-lab data in Table 7.6. All results were generated with passive NSSD forces. The algorithms A1-A4 are detailed in Section 7.5.

Dataset	Before registr.	Explicit scheme				FED			
		A1	A2	A3	A4	A1	A2	A3	A4
Case 01	3.892	1.243	1.258	1.265	1.204	1.216	1.181	1.176	1.160
Case 02	4.338	1.260	1.105	1.118	1.145	1.206	1.066	1.067	1.102
Case 03	6.943	1.727	1.292	1.296	1.348	1.586	1.253	1.252	1.276
Case 04	9.830	2.566	2.423	2.433	2.499	2.304	1.913	2.225	2.165
Case 05	7.477	2.201	1.532	1.657	1.573	2.205	1.501	1.553	1.524
Case 06	10.89	3.358	1.727	1.962	2.160	3.301	1.572	1.568	1.873
Case 07	11.03	5.989	2.523	3.797	3.911	5.558	2.012	2.293	3.522
Case 08	14.99	6.809	2.016	3.979	3.286	6.745	1.592	2.776	3.267
Case 09	7.918	2.478	1.676	1.934	1.819	2.225	1.556	1.693	1.554
Case 10	7.301	2.845	1.644	1.858	2.174	2.783	1.475	1.508	1.978
Average	8.461	3.048	1.720	2.130	2.112	2.913	1.512	1.711	1.942

List of Notations

Functions and sets

f	one-dimensional function, $f : \Omega \to \mathbb{R}$
$\boldsymbol{f}$	d-dimensional function, $\boldsymbol{f} : \Omega \to \mathbb{R}^d$ with $\boldsymbol{f} = (f_1, \ldots, f_d)^T$
M	Matrix
$\mathcal{J}$	Functional
$\mathcal{M}$	Evaluation metric, see Section 7.1.3
Ω, Σ	Open sets, with Σ generally denoting a subset of Ω
$\delta\Omega$	Boundary of set Ω
Γ	Boundary of Σ with $\Gamma := \delta\Sigma$
$\overline{\Omega}$	Closed set, $\overline{\Omega} = \Omega \cup \delta\Omega$

Images and image domains, see Appendix A

d	Dimension
Ω	Image domain, $\Omega \subset \mathbb{R}^d$
$\boldsymbol{x}$	Image coordinate vector, $\boldsymbol{x} \in \Omega$
I	Image, $I : \Omega \to \mathbb{R}$
R	Reference image
T	Template image
B	Baseline image
A	Atlas image
N	Number of discrete grid points, $N = N_1 \cdots N_d$
$\Omega^{\#}$	Set of discrete grid points, $\Omega^{\#} := \{\boldsymbol{x}_1, \ldots, \boldsymbol{x}_N\}$
$\boldsymbol{x}_j$	Discrete grid coordinate, $\boldsymbol{x}_j = (x_{j_1}, \ldots, x_{j_d})^T$, $j = 1, \ldots, N$
$\vec{I}$	Linearized discrete image vector, $\vec{I} := (I(\boldsymbol{x}_j))_{j=1,\ldots,N} \in \mathbb{R}^{N \times 1}$

Particular functions for registration, see Chapter 3

φ	Transformation, $\varphi : \Omega \to \Omega$
$\boldsymbol{u}$	Displacement field, $\boldsymbol{u} : \Omega \to \mathbb{R}^d$
$\boldsymbol{v}$	Velocity field, $\boldsymbol{v} : \Omega \to \mathbb{R}^d$
$\vec{U}$	Linearized displacement field, $\vec{U} := (\vec{U}_1, \ldots, \vec{U}_d)^T$

Particular functions for segmentation, see Chapter 4

ϕ	Level set function
ϕ_I	Level set function in image I
S_I	Binary segmentation in image I, $S_i : \Omega \to \{0,1\}$

Derivative operators

∂_t Partial derivative in direction t, $\partial_t := \frac{\partial}{\partial t}$

∇ Gradient $\nabla := (\partial_{x_1}, \ldots, \partial_{x_d})^T$

Δ Laplace operator $\Delta \boldsymbol{u} := (\Delta u_1, \ldots, \Delta u_d)^T$ with $\Delta u_l := \nabla \cdot \nabla u_l$

$\mathcal{H}(u)$ Hessian matrix $\mathcal{H}(\boldsymbol{u}) := \nabla \nabla^T u$

$\delta \mathcal{J}[\boldsymbol{u}; \boldsymbol{v}]$ Gâteaux derivative of $\mathcal{J}[\boldsymbol{u}]$ in direction $\boldsymbol{v}$, $\delta \mathcal{J}[\boldsymbol{u}; \boldsymbol{v}] := \langle \nabla \mathcal{J}[\boldsymbol{u}], \boldsymbol{v} \rangle_{L^2(\Omega)}$

Other operators

$\langle \cdot, \cdot \rangle$ L^2 inner product, $\langle \boldsymbol{u}, \boldsymbol{v} \rangle_{L^2(\Omega)} := \int_\Omega \boldsymbol{u}(\boldsymbol{x}) \cdot \boldsymbol{v}(\boldsymbol{x}) \, d\boldsymbol{x}$

$\| \cdot \|$ L^2 norm of a function, $\| \boldsymbol{u} \| := \int_\Omega \| \boldsymbol{u}(\boldsymbol{x}) \|^2 \, d\boldsymbol{x}$

$\| \cdot \|$ L^2 norm of a vector, $\| \boldsymbol{u}(\boldsymbol{x}) \| := \sqrt{\sum_{i=1}^d u_i(\boldsymbol{x})}$

$*$ Filter operation

$\otimes$ Kronecker product

Weights and parameters

τ Step size

α Regularization weight

μ, λ Linear-elastic parameters

β Weighting parameter of the joint framework

γ Weight of the gradient term

ω Weight for anisotropic diffusion and DDR

Bibliography

[ACS 2011] ACS, "Cancer Facts & Figures 2011". Tech. rep., American Cancer Society, 2011.

[Adalsteinsson and Sethian 1994] Adalsteinsson, D., Sethian, J. A. "A Fast Level Set Method for Propagating Interfaces". *J Comp Phys* 118, 269–277, 1994.

[Aljabar et al. 2009] Aljabar, P., Heckemann, R. A., Hammers, A., Hajnal, J. V., Rueckert, D. "Multi-atlas based segmentation of brain images: atlas selection and its effect on accuracy". *NeuroImage* 46 (3), 726–738, 2009.

[Amelon et al. 2012] Amelon, R. E., Cao, K., Reinhardt, J. M., Christensen, G. E., Raghavan, M. L., "Estimation of lung lobar sliding using image registration". In: Molthen, R. C., Weaver, J. B. (Eds.), Proc SPIE. p. 83171H, 2012.

[An et al. 2005] An, J.-h., Chen, Y., Huang, F., Wilson, D. C., Geiser, E. A., "A Variational PDE Based Level Set Method for a Simultaneous Segmentation and Non-rigid Registration". In: Duncan, J. S., Gerig, G. (Eds.), Med Image Comput Comput Assist Interv. pp. 286–293, 2005.

[Andresen and Nielsen 2001] Andresen, P. R., Nielsen, M. "Non-rigid registration by geometry-constrained diffusion". *Med Image Anal* 5 (2), 81–88, 2001.

[Armato and Sensakovic 2004] Armato, III, S. G., Sensakovic, W. F. "Automated Lung Segmentation for Thoracic CT: Impact on Computer-Aided Diagnosis". *Acad Radiol* 11 (9), 1011–1021, 2004.

[Arsigny 2006] Arsigny, V., "Processing Data in Lie Groups: An Algebraic Approach. Application to Non-Linear Registration and Diffusion Tensor MRI". Ph.D. thesis, l'École polytechnique, Palaiseau, France, 2006.

[Arsigny et al. 2006a] Arsigny, V., Commowick, O., Pennec, X., Ayache, N., "A Log-Euclidean Framework for Statistics on Diffeomorphisms". In: Larsen, R., Nielsen, M., Sporring, J. (Eds.), Med Image Comput Comput Assist Interv. LNCS 4191. pp. 924–931, 2006.

[Arsigny et al. 2006b] Arsigny, V., Commowick, O., Pennec, X., Ayache, N., "A Log-Euclidean Polyaffine Framework for Locally Rigid or Affine Registration". In: Pluim, J. P. W., Likar, B., Gerritsen, F. A. (Eds.), Biomedical Image Registration. LNCS 4057. pp. 120–127, 2006.

[Ashburner 2007] Ashburner, J. "A fast diffeomorphic image registration algorithm". *NeuroImage* 38 (1), 95–113, 2007.

[Ashburner and Friston 2005] Ashburner, J., Friston, K. J. "Unified segmentation". *NeuroImage* 26 (3), 839–851, 2005.

[Avants et al. 2008] Avants, B. B., Epstein, C. L., Grossman, M., Gee, J. C. "Symmetric Diffeomorphic Image Registration with Cross-Correlation: Evaluating Automated Labeling of Elderly and Neurodegenerative Brain". *Med Image Anal* 12 (1), 26–41, 2008.

[Avants et al. 2006] Avants, B. B., Schoenemann, P. T., Gee, J. C. "Lagrangian frame diffeomorphic image registration: Morphometric comparison of human and chimpanzee cortex". *Med Image Anal* 10 (3), 397–412, 2006.

[Avants et al. 2012] Avants, B. B., Tustison, N. J., Song, G., Wu, B., Stauffer, M., McCormick, M. M., Johnson, H. J., Gee, J. C., "A Unified Image Registration Framework for ITK". In: Dawant, B. M., Christensen, G. E., Fitzpatrick, J. M., Rueckert, D. (Eds.), Biomedical Image Registration. LNCS 7359. pp. 266–275, 2012.

[Aziz et al. 2004] Aziz, A., Ashizawa, K., Nagaoki, K., Hayashi, K. "High Resolution CT Anatomy of the Pulmonary Fissures". *J Thorac Imaging* 19 (3), 186–191, 2004.

[Beg et al. 2005] Beg, M. F., Miller, M. I., Trouvé, A., Younes, L. "Computing large deformation metric mappings via geodesic flows of diffeomorphisms". *Int J Comput Vis* 61 (2), 139–157, 2005.

[Besl and McKay 1992] Besl, P. J., McKay, H. D. "A method for registration of 3-D shapes". *IEEE Trans Pattern Anal Mach Intell* 14 (2), 239–256, 1992.

[Beuthien et al. 2010] Beuthien, B., Kamen, A., Fischer, B., "Recursive Green's Function Registration". In: Jiang, T., Navab, N., Pluim, J. P. W., Viergever, M. A. (Eds.), Med Image Comput Comput Assist Interv. LNCS 6362. pp. 546–553, 2010.

[Bookstein 1989] Bookstein, F. L. "Principal warps: thin-plate splines and the decomposition of deformations". *IEEE Trans Pattern Anal Mach Intell* 11 (6), 567–585, 1989.

[Bossa et al. 2008] Bossa, M. N., Zacur, E., Olmos, S., "Algorithms for computing the group exponential of diffeomorphisms: Performance evaluation". In: Proc IEEE Comput Soc Conf Comput Vis Pattern Recognit. pp. 1–8, 2008.

[Briggs et al. 2000] Briggs, W. L., Henson, V. E., McComick, S. F., "A Multigrid Tutorial", 2nd Edition. SIAM: Society for Industrial and Applied Mathematics, 2000.

[Bro-Nielsen and Gramkow 1996] Bro-Nielsen, M., Gramkow, C., "Fast Fluid Registration of Medical Images". In: Höhne, K. H., Kikinis, R. (Eds.), Conference on Visualization in Biomedical Computing. LNCS 1131. pp. 265–276, 1996.

[Brock et al. 2010] Brock, K. K., et al. "Results of a multi-institution deformable registration accuracy study (MIDRAS)". *Int J Radiat Oncol Biol Phys* 76 (2), 583–596, 2010.

[Broit 1981] Broit, C., "Optimal registration of deformed images ". Ph.D. thesis, University of Pennsylvania, 1981.

[Brown 1992] Brown, L. G. "A survey of image registration techniques". *ACM Comput Surv* 24 (4), 325–376, 1992.

[Brox et al. 2004] Brox, T., Bruhn, A., Papenberg, N., Weickert, J., "High Accuracy Optical Flow Estimation Based on a Theory for Warping". In: Pajdla, T., Matas, J. (Eds.), Europ Conf Comp Vis. pp. 25–36, 2004.

[Brox and Weickert 2004] Brox, T., Weickert, J., "Level Set Based Image Segmentation with Multiple Regions". In: Rasmussen, C. E., Bülthoff, H. H., Schölkopf, B., Giese, M. A. (Eds.), Pattern Recognit. LNCS 3175. pp. 415–423, 2004.

[Buzug 2008] Buzug, T. M., "Computed Tomography - From Photon Statistics to Modern Cone-Beam CT". Springer, Berlin, Heidelberg, 2008.

[Cao et al. 2010a] Cao, K., Ding, K., Christensen, G. E., Raghavan, M. L., Amelon, R. E., Reinhardt, J. M., "Unifying Vascular Information in Intensity-Based Nonrigid Lung CT Registration". In: Fischer, B., Dawant, B. M., Lorenz, C. (Eds.), Biomedical Image Registration. LNCS 6204. pp. 1–12, 2010.

[Cao et al. 2010b] Cao, K., Du, K., Ding, K., Reinhardt, J. M., Christensen, G. E., "Regularized Nonrigid Registration of Lung CT Images by Preserving Tissue Volume and Vesselness Measure". In: van Ginneken, B., Murphy, K., Heimann, T., Pekar, V., Deng, X. (Eds.), Medical Image Analysis for the Clinic: A Grand Challenge, MICCAI 2010. pp. 43–54, 2010.

[Caselles et al. 1993] Caselles, V., Catté, F., Coll, T., Dibos, F. "A geometric model for active contours in image processing". *Numer Math* 66 (1), 1–31, 1993.

[Caselles et al. 1997] Caselles, V., Kimmel, R., Sapiro, G. "Geodesic Active Contours". *Int J Comput Vis* 22 (1), 61–79, 1997.

[Castillo et al. 2010a] Castillo, E., Castillo, R., Martinez, J., Shenoy, M., Guerrero, T. "Four-dimensional deformable image registration using trajectory modeling". *Phys Med Biol* 55 (1), 305–327, 2010.

[Castillo et al. 2012] Castillo, E., Castillo, R., White, B., Rojo, J., Guerrero, T. "Least median of squares filtering of locally optimal point matches for compressible flow image registration". *Phys Med Biol* 57 (15), 4827–4833, 2012.

[Castillo et al. 2009] Castillo, R., Castillo, E., Guerra, R., Johnson, V. E., McPhail, T., Garg, A. K., Guerrero, T. "A framework for evaluation of deformable image registration spatial accuracy using large landmark point sets". *Phys Med Biol* 54, 1849–1870, 2009.

[Castillo et al. 2010b] Castillo, R., Castillo, E., Martinez, J., Guerrero, T. "Ventilation from four-dimensional computed tomography: density versus Jacobian methods". *Phys Med Biol* 55 (16), 4661–4685, 2010.

[Chan and Vese 2001] Chan, T. F., Vese, L. A. "Active contours without edges". *IEEE Trans Image Process* 10 (2), 266–277, 2001.

[Christensen 1994] Christensen, G. E., "Deformable shape models for anatomy". Ph.D. thesis, Washington University, 1994.

[Christensen and Johnson 2001] Christensen, G. E., Johnson, H. J. "Consistent image registration". *IEEE Trans Med Imag* 20 (7), 568–582, 2001.

[Christensen et al. 1996] Christensen, G. E., Rabbitt, R. D., Miller, M. I. "Deformable templates using large deformation kinematics". *IEEE Trans Image Process* 5 (10), 1435–1447, 1996.

[Clarenz et al. 2006] Clarenz, U., Droske, M., Henn, S., Rumpf, M., Witsch, K., "Computational Methods for Nonlinear Image Registration". In: Scherzer, O. (Ed.), Mathematical Models for Registration and Applications to Medical Imaging. Springer, Berlin, Heidelberg, pp. 81–106, 2006.

[Commowick et al. 2008] Commowick, O., Arsigny, V., Isambert, A., Costa, J., Dhermain, F., Bidault, F., Bondiau, P., Ayache, N., Malandain, G. "An efficient locally affine framework for the smooth registration of anatomical structures". *Med Image Anal* 12 (4), 427–441, 2008.

[Cremers et al. 2007] Cremers, D., Fluck, O., Rousson, M., Aharon, S., "A Probabilistic Level Set Formulation for Interactive Organ Segmentation". In: Pluim, J. P. W., Reinhardt, J. M. (Eds.), Proc SPIE. p. 65120V, 2007.

[Crum et al. 2005] Crum, W. R., Tanner, C., Hawkes, D. J. "Anisotropic multi-scale fluid registration: evaluation in magnetic resonance breast imaging". *Phys Med Biol* 50 (21), 5153–5174, 2005.

[Datteri and Dawant 2012] Datteri, R. D., Dawant, B. M., "Estimation and Reduction of Target Registration Error". In: Ayache, N., Delingette, H., Golland, P., Mori, K. (Eds.), Med Image Comput Comput Assist Interv. LNCS 7512. pp. 139–146, 2012.

[Davis et al. 1997] Davis, M. H., Khotanzad, A., Flamig, D. P., Harms, S. E. "A physics-based coordinate transformation for 3-D image matching". *IEEE Trans Med Imag* 16 (3), 317–328, 1997.

[Delingette 1999] Delingette, H. "General object reconstruction based on simplex meshes". *Int J Comput Vis* 32 (2), 111–142, 1999.

[Delmon et al. 2011] Delmon, V., Rit, S., Pinho, R., Sarrut, D., "Direction dependent B-splines decomposition for the registration of sliding objects". In: Beichel, R., de Bruijne, M., van Ginneken, B., Kabus, S., Kiraly, A., Kuhnigk, J. M., McClelland, J. R., Mori, K., van Rikxoort, E. M., Rit, S. (Eds.), Fourth International Workshop on Pulmonary Image Analysis, MICCAI 2011. pp. 45–55, 2011.

[Deriche 1987] Deriche, R. "Using Canny's criteria to derive a recursively implemented optimal edge detector". *Int J Comput Vis* 1 (2), 167–187, 1987.

[Ding et al. 2009] Ding, K., Yin, Y., Cao, K., Christensen, G. E., Lin, C.-L., Hoffman, E. A., Reinhardt, J. M., "Evaluation of Lobar Biomechanics during Respiration Using Image Registration". In: Yang, G.-Z., Hawkes, D. J., Rueckert, D., Noble, J. A., Taylor, C. (Eds.), Med Image Comput Comput Assist Interv. LNCS 5761. pp. 739–746, 2009.

[Doel et al. 2012] Doel, T., Matin, T. N., Gleeson, F. V., Gavaghan, D. J., Grau, V., "Pulmonary lobe segmentation from CT images using fissureness, airways, vessels and multilevel B-splines". In: Proc IEEE Int Symp Biomed Imaging. pp. 1491–1494, 2012.

[Droske and Rumpf 2007] Droske, M., Rumpf, M. "Multiscale Joint Segmentation and Registration of Image Morphology". *IEEE Trans Pattern Anal Mach Intell* 29 (12), 2181–2194, 2007.

[Dupuis et al. 1998] Dupuis, P., Grenander, U., Miller, M. I. "Variational Problems on Flows of Diffeomorphisms for Image Matching". *Q Appl Math* LVI (3), 1998.

[Ehrhardt et al. 2007] Ehrhardt, J., Werner, R., Saering, D., Lu, W., Low, D. A., Handels, H. "An optical flow based method for improved reconstruction of 4D CT data sets acquired during free breathing". *Med Phys* 34 (2), 711–721, 2007.

[Ehrhardt et al. 2010] Ehrhardt, J., Werner, R., Schmidt-Richberg, A., Handels, H., "Automatic Landmark Detection and Non-linear Landmark- and Surface-based Registration of Lung CT Images". In: van Ginneken, B., Murphy, K., Heimann, T., Pekar, V., Deng, X. (Eds.), Medical Image Analysis for the Clinic: A Grand Challenge, MICCAI 2010. pp. 165–174, 2010.

[Ehrhardt et al. 2011] Ehrhardt, J., Werner, R., Schmidt-Richberg, A., Handels, H. "Statistical modeling of 4D respiratory lung motion using diffeomorphic image registration". *IEEE Trans Med Imag* 30 (2), 251–265, 2011.

[Ens et al. 2008] Ens, K., von Berg, J., Kabus, S., Lorenz, C., Fischer, B., "A unified framework for joint registration and segmentation". In: Reinhardt, J. M., Pluim, J. P. W. (Eds.), Proc SPIE. p. 691406, 2008.

[Ezhil et al. 2008] Ezhil, M., Choi, B., Starkschall, G., Bucci, M. K., Vedam, S., Balter, P. "Comparison of Rigid and Adaptive Methods of Propagating Gross Tumor Volume Through Respiratory Phases of Four-Dimensional Computed Tomography Image Data Set". *Int J Radiat Oncol Biol Phys* 71 (1), 290–296, 2008.

[Fischer and Modersitzki 1999] Fischer, B., Modersitzki, J. "Fast inversion of matrices arising in image processing". *Numer Algorithm* 22 (1), 1–11, 1999.

[Fischer and Modersitzki 2002] Fischer, B., Modersitzki, J. "Fast diffusion registration". *Contemp Math* 313, 117–127, 2002.

[Fischer and Modersitzki 2004] Fischer, B., Modersitzki, J. "A unified approach to fast image registration and a new curvature based registration technique". *Lin Algebra Appl* 380, 107–124, 2004.

[Fitzpatrick and West 2001] Fitzpatrick, J. M., West, J. B. "The distribution of target registration error in rigid-body point-based registration". *IEEE Trans Med Imag* 20 (9), 917–927, 2001.

[Flach and Schlesinger 2002] Flach, B., Schlesinger, D., "Unifying Registration and Segmentation for Multi-Sensor Images". In: Van Gool, L. (Ed.), Pattern Recognit. LNCS 2449. pp. 190–197, 2002.

[Forkert et al. 2012] Forkert, N. D., Schmidt-Richberg, A., Fiehler, J., Illies, T., Möller, D., Säring, D., Handels, H., Ehrhardt, J. "3D cerebrovascular segmentation combining fuzzy vessel enhancement and level-sets with anisotropic energy weights". *Magn Reson Imaging*, 2012. In Press.

[Frangi et al. 1998] Frangi, A. F., Niessen, W. J., Vincken, K. L., Viergever, M. A., "Multiscale Vessel Enhancement Filtering". In: Wells, III, W. M., Colchester, A., Delp, S. (Eds.), Med Image Comput Comput Assist Interv. LNCS 1496. pp. 130–137, 1998.

[Freiman et al. 2011] Freiman, M., Voss, S. D., Warfield, S. K., "Demons registration with local affine adaptive regularization: application to registration of abdominal structures". In: Proc IEEE Int Symp Biomed Imaging. pp. 1219–1222, 2011.

[Frohn-Schauf et al. 2007] Frohn-Schauf, C., Henn, S., Witsch, K. "Multigrid based total variation image registration". *Comput Visual Sci* 11 (2), 101–113, 2007.

[Garcia et al. 2010] Garcia, V., Vercauteren, T., Malandain, G., Ayache, N., "Diffeomorphic demons and the EMPIRE10 challenge". In: van Ginneken, B., Murphy, K., Heimann, T., Pekar, V., Deng, X. (Eds.), Medical Image Analysis for the Clinic: A Grand Challenge, MICCAI 2010. pp. 91–98, 2010.

[Gentzsch 1980] Gentzsch, W., "Numerical solution of linear and non-linear parabolic differential equations by a time-discretisation of third order accuracy". In: Hirschel, E. H. (Ed.), Conference on Numerical Methods in Fluid Mechanics. pp. 109–117, 1980.

[Gerschgorin 1931] Gerschgorin, S. "Über die Abgrenzung der Eigenwerte einer Matrix". *Izvestija Akademii Nauk SSSR, Serija Matematika* 7 (3), 749–754, 1931.

[Gorbunova et al. 2010] Gorbunova, V., Jacobs, S. S. A. M., Lo, P., Dirksen, A., Nielsen, M., Bab-Hadiashar, A., de Bruijne, M., "Early Detection of Emphysema Progression". In: Jiang, T., Navab, N., Pluim, J. P. W., Viergever, M. A. (Eds.), Med Image Comput Comput Assist Interv. LNCS 6362. pp. 193–200, 2010.

[Gorbunova et al. 2012] Gorbunova, V., Sporring, J., Lo, P., Loeve, M., Tiddens, H. A., Nielsen, M., Dirksen, A., de Bruijne, M. "Mass preserving image registration for lung CT". *Med Image Anal* 16 (4), 786–795, 2012.

[Goshtasby 2012a] Goshtasby, A. A., "Image Registration". Advances in Computer Vision and Pattern Recognition. Springer, London, 2012.

[Goshtasby 2012b] Goshtasby, A. A., "Similarity and Dissimilarity Measures". In: Image Registration. Springer, London, pp. 7–66, 2012.

[Grewenig et al. 2010] Grewenig, S., Weickert, J., Bruhn, A., "From Box Filtering to Fast Explicit Diffusion". In: Goesele, M., Roth, S., Kuijper, A., Schiele, B., Schindler, K. (Eds.), Pattern Recognit. LNCS 6376. pp. 533–542, 2010.

[Guimond et al. 1998] Guimond, A., Meunier, J., Thirion, J.-P., "Automatic Computation of Average Brain Models". In: Wells, III, W. M., Colchester, A., Delp, S. (Eds.), Med Image Comput Comput Assist Interv. LNCS 1496. pp. 631–640, 1998.

[Gwosdek et al. 2010] Gwosdek, P., Zimmer, H., Grewenig, S., Bruhn, A., Weickert, J., "A highly efficient GPU implementation for variational optic flow based on the Euler-Lagrange framework". Tech. Rep. 267, Universität des Saarlandes, 2010.

[Haber and Modersitzki 2006] Haber, E., Modersitzki, J., "Intensity Gradient Based Registration and Fusion of Multi-modal Images". In: Larsen, R., Nielsen, M., Sporring, J. (Eds.), Med Image Comput Comput Assist Interv. LNCS 4191. pp. 726–733, 2006.

[Hajnal et al. 2001] Hajnal, J. V., Hill, D. L. G., Hawkes, D. J., "Medical Image Registration". CRC Press, 2001.

[Han 2010] Han, X., "Feature-constrained Nonlinear Registration of Lung CT Images". In: van Ginneken, B., Murphy, K., Heimann, T., Pekar, V., Deng, X. (Eds.), Medical Image Analysis for the Clinic: A Grand Challenge, MICCAI 2010. pp. 63–72, 2010.

[Hayashi et al. 2001] Hayashi, K., Aziz, A., Ashizawa, K., Hayashi, H., Nagaoki, K., Otsuji, H. "Radiographic and CT appearances of the major fissures". *Radiographics* 21 (4), 861–874, 2001.

[Heath et al. 2007] Heath, E., Collins, D. L., Keall, P. J., Dong, L., Seuntjens, J. "Quantification of accuracy of the automated nonlinear image matching and anatomical labeling (ANIMAL) nonlinear registration algorithm for 4D CT images of lung". *Med Phys* 34 (11), 4409–4421, 2007.

[Heinrich et al. 2012] Heinrich, M. P., Jenkinson, M., Brady, M., Schnabel, J. A., "Globally Optimal Deformable Registration on a Minimum Spanning Tree Using Dense Displacement Sampling". In: Ayache, N., Delingette, H., Golland, P., Mori, K. (Eds.), Med Image Comput Comput Assist Interv. LNCS 7512. pp. 115–122, 2012.

[Heldmann 2006] Heldmann, S., "Non-Linear Registration Based on Mutual Information". Ph.D. thesis, University of Lübeck, 2006.

[Hermosillo et al. 2002] Hermosillo, G., Chefd'Hotel, C., Faugeras, O. D. "Variational Methods for Multimodal Image Matching". *Int J Comput Vis* 50 (3), 329–343, 2002.

[Hernandez et al. 2009] Hernandez, M., Bossa, M. N., Olmos, S. "Registration of Anatomical Images Using Paths of Diffeomorphisms Parameterized with Stationary Vector Field Flows". *Int J Comput Vis* 85 (3), 291–306, 2009.

[Hill et al. 2001] Hill, D. L. G., Batchelor, P. G., Holden, M., Hawkes, D. J. "Medical image registration". *Phys Med Biol* 46 (3), R1–45, 2001.

[Hoffman et al. 2004] Hoffman, E. A., Clough, A. V., Christensen, G. E., Lin, C.-L., McLennan, G., Reinhardt, J. M., Simon, B. A., Sonka, M., Tawhai, M. H., van Beek, E. J. R., Wang, G. "The comprehensive imaging-based analysis of the lung: a forum for team science". *Acad Radiol* 11 (12), 1370–1380, 2004.

[Horn and Schunck 1981] Horn, B. K. P., Schunck, B. G. "Determining Optical Flow". *Artiff Intell* 16 (1-3), 185–203, 1981.

[Hu et al. 2001] Hu, S., Hoffman, E. A., Reinhardt, J. M. "Automatic Lung Segmentation for Accurate Quantitation of Volumetric X-Ray CT Images". *IEEE Trans Med Imag* 20 (6), 490–498, 2001.

[Hufnagel et al. 2009] Hufnagel, H., Ehrhardt, J., Pennec, X., Schmidt-Richberg, A., Handels, H., "Level Set Segmentation Using a Point-Based Statistical Shape Model Relying on Correspondence Probabilities". In: Pohl, K. M., Joshi, S., Wells, III, W. M. (Eds.), Workshop Probabilistic Models for Medical Image Analysis, PMMIA 09, Workshop proceedings from MICCAI 2009. pp. 34–44, 2009.

[ICRU 1999] ICRU, "Report 62: Prescribing, Recording and Reporting Photon Beam Therapy (Supplement to ICRU Report 50)". Tech. Rep. 62, ICRU, 1999.

[ICRU 2010] ICRU. "Report 83: Prescribing, Recording, and Reporting Photon-Beam Intensity-Modulated Radiation Therapy (IMRT)". *Journal of the ICRU* 10 (1), 1–106, 2010.

[Kabus 2006] Kabus, S., "Multiple-Material Variational Image Registration". Ph.D. thesis, University of Lübeck, 2006.

[Kabus et al. 2006] Kabus, S., Franz, A., Fischer, B., "Variational image registration with local properties". In: Pluim, J. P. W., Likar, B., Gerritsen, F. A. (Eds.), Biomedical Image Registration. LNCS 4057. pp. 92–100, 2006.

[Kabus et al. 2009] Kabus, S., Klinder, T., Murphy, K., van Ginneken, B., Lorenz, C., Pluim, J. P. W., "Evaluation of 4D-CT Lung Registration". In: Yang, G.-Z., Hawkes, D. J., Rueckert, D., Noble, J. A., Taylor, C. (Eds.), Med Image Comput Comput Assist Interv. LNCS 5761. pp. 747–754, 2009.

[Kabus and Lorenz 2010] Kabus, S., Lorenz, C., "Fast Elastic Image Registration". In: van Ginneken, B., Murphy, K., Heimann, T., Pekar, V., Deng, X. (Eds.), Medical Image Analysis for the Clinic: A Grand Challenge, MICCAI 2010. pp. 81–89, 2010.

[Kalender 2011] Kalender, W. A., "Computed Tomography", 3rd Edition. Wiley, 2011.

[Kass et al. 1987] Kass, M., Witkin, A., Terzopoulos, D. "Snakes: Active Contour Models". *Int J Comput Vis* 1 (4), 321–331, 1987.

[Keall et al. 2006] Keall, P. J., Mageras, G. S., Balter, J. M., Emery, R. S., Forster, K., Jiang, S. B., Kapatoes, J. M., Low, D. A., Murphy, M. J., Murray, B. R., Ramsey, C. R., van Herk, M. B., Vedam, S. S., Wong, J. W., Yorke, E. "The management of respiratory motion in radiation oncology report of AAPM Task Group 76". *Med Phys* 33 (10), 3874–3900, 2006.

[Kim and Fessler 2004] Kim, J., Fessler, J. A. "Intensity-Based Image Registration Using Robust Correlation Coefficients". *IEEE Trans Med Imag* 23 (11), 1430–1444, 2004.

[Kiriyanthan et al. 2012] Kiriyanthan, S., Fundana, K., Cattin, P., "Discontinuity Preserving Registration of Abdominal MR Images with Apparent Sliding Organ Motion". In: Yoshida, H., Sakas, G., Linguraru, M. G. (Eds.), Abdominal Imaging 2011. LNCS 7601. pp. 231–239, 2012.

[Klein et al. 2010] Klein, S., Staring, M., Murphy, K., Viergever, M. A., Pluim, J. P. W. "elastix: a toolbox for intensity-based medical image registration". *IEEE Trans Med Imag* 29 (1), 196–205, 2010.

[Lassen et al. 2010] Lassen, B., Kuhnigk, J.-M., Friman, O., Krass, S., Peitgen, H.-O., "Automatic Segmentation of Lung Lobes in CT Images Based on Fissures, Vessels, and Bronchi". In: Proc IEEE Int Symp Biomed Imaging. pp. 560–563, 2010.

[Li et al. 2012] Li, B., Christensen, G. E., Hoffman, E. A., McLennan, G., Reinhardt, J. M. "Establishing a Normative Atlas of the Human Lung: Computing the Average Transformation and Atlas Construction". *Acad Radiol* 19 (11), 1368–1381, 2012.

[Li et al. 2010] Li, C., Xu, C., Gui, C., Fox, M. D. "Distance Regularized Level Set Evolution and its Application to Image Segmentation". *IEEE Trans Image Process* 19 (12), 3243–3254, 2010.

[Lindeberg 1990] Lindeberg, T. "Scale-Space for Discrete Signals". *IEEE Trans Pattern Anal Mach Intell* 13 (3), 234–254, 1990.

[Loeckx et al. 2004] Loeckx, D., Maes, F., Vandermeulen, D., Suetens, P., "Nonrigid Image Registration Using Free-Form Deformations with a Local Rigidity Constraint". In: Barillot, C., Haynor, D. R., Hellier, P. (Eds.), Med Image Comput Comput Assist Interv. LNCS 3216. pp. 639–646, 2004.

[Lorensen and Cline 1987] Lorensen, W. E., Cline, H. E. "Marching cubes: A high resolution 3D surface construction algorithm". *ACM SIGGRAPH Computer Graphics* 21 (4), 163–169, 1987.

[Low et al. 2003] Low, D. A., Nystrom, M., Kalinin, E., Parikh, P., Dempsey, J. F., Bradley, J. D., Mutic, S., Wahab, S. H., Islam, T., Christensen, G. E., Politte, D. G., Whiting, B. R. "A method for the reconstruction of four-dimensional synchronized CT scans acquired during free breathing". *Med Phys* 30 (6), 1254–1263, 2003.

[Lu et al. 2011] Lu, C., Chelikani, S., Papademetris, X., Knisely, J. P., Milosevic, M. F., Chen, Z., Jaffray, D. A., Staib, L. H., Duncan, J. S. "An integrated approach to segmentation and nonrigid registration for application in image-guided pelvic radiotherapy". *Med Image Anal* 15 (5), 772–785, 2011.

[Lu et al. 2004] Lu, W., Chen, M.-L., Olivera, G. H., Ruchala, K. J., Mackie, T. R. "Fast free-form deformable registration via calculus of variations". *Phys Med Biol* 49 (14), 3067–3087, 2004.

[Maes et al. 1997] Maes, F., Collignon, A., Vandermeulen, D., Marchal, G., Suetens, P. "Multimodality image registration by maximization of mutual information". *IEEE Trans Med Imag* 16 (2), 187–198, 1997.

[Mageras and Yorke 2004] Mageras, G. S., Yorke, E. "Deep inspiration breath hold and respiratory gating strategies for reducing organ motion in radiation treatment". *Semin Radiat Oncol* 14 (1), 65–75, 2004.

[Maintz and Viergever 1998] Maintz, J. B. A., Viergever, M. A. "A survey of medical image registration". *Med Image Anal* 2 (1), 1–36, 1998.

[Malladi et al. 1995] Malladi, R., Sethian, J. A., Vemuri, B. C. "Shape Modeling with Front Propagation: A Level Set Approach". *IEEE Trans Pattern Anal Mach Intell* 17 (2), 158–175, 1995.

[McNitt-Gray 2004] McNitt-Gray, M. F., "Tradeoffs in CT Image Quality and Dose". In: AAPM 46th Annual Meeting, 2004.

[Messay et al. 2010] Messay, T., Hardie, R. C., Rogers, S. K. "A New Computationally Efficient CAD System for Pulmonary Nodule Detection in CT Imagery". *Med Image Anal*, 2010.

[Modat et al. 2010a] Modat, M., McClelland, J. R., Ourselin, S., "Lung registration using the NiftyReg package". In: van Ginneken, B., Murphy, K., Heimann, T., Pekar, V., Deng, X. (Eds.), Medical Image Analysis for the Clinic: A Grand Challenge, MICCAI 2010. pp. 33–42, 2010.

[Modat et al. 2010b] Modat, M., Ridgway, G. R., Taylor, Z. A., Lehmann, M., Barnes, J., Hawkes, D. J., Fox, N. C., Ourselin, S. "Fast free-form deformation using graphics processing units". *Comput Methods Programs Biomed* 98 (3), 278–284, 2010.

[Modersitzki 2004] Modersitzki, J., "Numerical Methods for Image Registration". Oxford University Press, 2004.

[Modersitzki 2009] Modersitzki, J., "FAIR: Flexible Algorithms for Image Registration". Fundamentals of Algorithms. SIAM: Society for Industrial and Applied Mathematics, 2009.

[Muenzing et al. 2012a] Muenzing, S. E. A., van Ginneken, B., Murphy, K., Pluim, J. P. W. "Supervised quality assessment of medical image registration: Application to intra-patient CT lung registration". *Med Image Anal*, 2012.

[Muenzing et al. 2010] Muenzing, S. E. A., van Ginneken, B., Pluim, J. P. W., "Knowledge Driven Regularization of the Deformation Field for PDE Based Non-Rigid Registration Algorithms". In: van Ginneken, B., Murphy, K., Heimann, T., Pekar, V., Deng, X. (Eds.), Medical Image Analysis for the Clinic: A Grand Challenge, MICCAI 2010. pp. 127–136, 2010.

[Muenzing et al. 2012b] Muenzing, S. E. A., van Ginneken, B., Pluim, J. P. W., "On Combining Algorithms for Deformable Image Registration". In: Dawant, B. M., Christensen, G. E., Fitzpatrick, J. M., Rueckert, D. (Eds.), Biomedical Image Registration. LNCS 7359. pp. 256–265, 2012.

[Murphy et al. 2011a] Murphy, K., van Ginneken, B., Klein, S., Staring, M., de Hoop, B. J., Viergever, M. A., Pluim, J. P. W. "Semi-automatic Construction of Reference Standards for Evaluation of Image Registration". *Med Image Anal* 15 (1), 71–84, 2011.

[Murphy et al. 2011b] Murphy, K., van Ginneken, B., Reinhardt, J. M., Kabus, S., Ding, K., Deng, X., et al. "Evaluation of Registration Methods on Thoracic CT: The EMPIRE10 Challenge". *IEEE Trans Med Imag* 30 (11), 1901–1920, 2011.

[Nagel and Enkelmann 1986] Nagel, H.-H., Enkelmann, W. "An Investigation of Smoothness Constraints for the Estimation of Displacement Vector Fields from Image
Sequences". *IEEE Trans Pattern Anal Mach Intell* PAMI-8 (5), 565–593, 1986.

[Nocedal and Wright 2006] Nocedal, J., Wright, S. J., "Numerical Optimization", 2nd
Edition. Springer, 2006.

[Noe et al. 2008] Noe, K. Ø., Tanderup, K., Lindegaard, J. C., Grau, C., Sørensen,
T. S. "GPU accelerated viscous-fluid deformable registration for radiotherapy". *Stud
Health Technol Inform* 132, 327–332, 2008.

[Nyúl et al. 2000] Nyúl, L. G., Udupa, J. K., Zhang, X. "New variants of a method of
MRI scale standardization". *IEEE Trans Med Imag* 19 (2), 143–150, 2000.

[Olesch et al. 2009] Olesch, J., Papenberg, N., Lange, T., Conrad, M., Fischer, B.,
"Matching CT and ultrasound data of the liver by landmark constrained image
registration". In: Miga, M. I., Wong, K. H. (Eds.), Proc SPIE. p. 72610G, 2009.

[Oliveira and Tavares 2012] Oliveira, F. P. M., Tavares, J. M. R. S. "Medical image
registration: a review". *Comput Methods Biomech Biomed Engin*, 1–21, 2012.

[Osher and Sethian 1988] Osher, S., Sethian, J. A. "Fronts Propagating with Curvature-
Dependent Speed: Algorithms Based on Hamilton-Jacobi Formulations". *J Comp
Phys* 79, 12–49, 1988.

[Pace et al. 2011] Pace, D. F., Enquobahrie, A., Yang, H., Aylward, S. R., Niethammer,
M., "Deformable Image Registration of Sliding Organs Using Anisotropic Diffusive
Regularization". In: Proc IEEE Int Symp Biomed Imaging. pp. 407–413, 2011.

[Paragios 2003] Paragios, N. "A level set approach for shape-driven segmentation and
tracking of the left ventricle". *IEEE Trans Med Imag* 22 (6), 773–776, 2003.

[Paragios and Deriche 2000] Paragios, N., Deriche, R., "Coupled Geodesic Active Regions
for Image Segmentation: A Level Set Approach". In: Vernon, D. (Ed.), Europ Conf
Comp Vis. pp. 224–240, 2000.

[Parzen 1962] Parzen, E. "On the estimation of a probability density function and
mode". *Ann Math Stat* 33, 1065–1076, 1962.

[Pennec 2006] Pennec, X. "Intrinsic Statistics on Riemannian Manifolds: Basic Tools
for Geometric Measurements". *J Math Imag Vis* 25 (1), 127–154, 2006.

[Pennec et al. 1999] Pennec, X., Cachier, P., Ayache, N., "Understanding the "Demon's
Algorithm": 3D Non-rigid Registration by Gradient Descent". In: Goos, G., Hartma-
nis, J., Leeuwen, J., Taylor, C., Colchester, A. (Eds.), Med Image Comput Comput
Assist Interv. pp. 597–605, 1999.

[Pennec et al. 2005] Pennec, X., Stefanescu, R., Arsigny, V., Fillard, P., Ayache, N., "Riemannian elasticity: A statistical regularization framework for non-linear registration". In: Duncan, J. S., Gerig, G. (Eds.), Med Image Comput Comput Assist Interv. pp. 943–950, 2005.

[Peroni et al. 2011] Peroni, M., Golland, P., Sharp, G. C., Baroni, G., "Ranking of Stopping Criteria for Log Domain Diffeomorphic Demons Application in Clinical Radiation Therapy". In: Conf Proc IEEE Eng Med Biol Soc. pp. 4884–4887, 2011.

[Pitiot and Guimond 2007] Pitiot, A., Guimond, A. "Geometrical regularization of displacement fields for histological image registration". Med Image Anal 12 (1), 16–25, 2007.

[Pohl et al. 2006] Pohl, K. M., Fisher, J., Grimson, W. E. L., Kikinis, R. "A Bayesian model for joint segmentation and registration". NeuroImage 31 (1), 228–239, 2006.

[Pu et al. 2009] Pu, J., Zheng, B., Leader, J. K., Fuhrman, C., Knollmann, F., Klym, A., Gur, D. "Pulmonary Lobe Segmentation in CT Examinations Using Implicit Surface Fitting". IEEE Trans Med Imag 28 (12), 1986–1996, 2009.

[Reinhardt et al. 2008] Reinhardt, J. M., Ding, K., Cao, K., Christensen, G. E., Hoffman, E. A., Bodas, S. V. "Registration-based estimates of local lung tissue expansion compared to xenon CT measures of specific ventilation". Med Image Anal 12 (6), 752–763, 2008.

[Rey et al. 2002] Rey, D., Subsol, G., Delingette, H., Ayache, N. "Automatic detection and segmentation of evolving processes in 3D medical images: Application to multiple sclerosis". Med Image Anal 6 (2), 163–179, 2002.

[Risser et al. 2011] Risser, L., Baluwala, H., Schnabel, J. A., "Diffeomorphic registration with sliding conditions: Application to the registration of lungs CT images". In: Beichel, R., de Bruijne, M., van Ginneken, B., Kabus, S., Kiraly, A., Kuhnigk, J. M., McClelland, J. R., Mori, K., van Rikxoort, E. M., Rit, S. (Eds.), Fourth International Workshop on Pulmonary Image Analysis, MICCAI 2011. pp. 79–90, 2011.

[Ross et al. 2010] Ross, J. C., San José Estépar, R., Kindlmann, G., Díaz, A., Westin, C.-F., Silverman, E. K., Washko, G. R., "Automatic Lung Lobe Segmentation Using Particles, Thin Plate Splines, and Maximum a Posteriori Estimation". In: Jiang, T., Navab, N., Pluim, J. P. W., Viergever, M. A. (Eds.), Med Image Comput Comput Assist Interv. pp. 163–171, 2010.

[Ruan et al. 2009] Ruan, D., Esedoglu, S., Fessler, J. A., "Discriminative sliding preserving regularization in medical image registration". In: Proc IEEE Int Symp Biomed Imaging. pp. 430–433, 2009.

[Rudin et al. 1992] Rudin, L. I., Osher, S., Fatemi, E. "Nonlinear total variation based noise removal algorithms". *Physica D* 60 (1-4), 259–268, 1992.

[Rueckert et al. 2006] Rueckert, D., Aljabar, P., Heckemann, R. A., Hajnal, J. V., Hammers, A., "Diffeomorphic Registration Using B-Splines". In: Larsen, R., Nielsen, M., Sporring, J. (Eds.), Med Image Comput Comput Assist Interv. LNCS 4191. pp. 702–709, 2006.

[Rueckert et al. 1999] Rueckert, D., Sonoda, L. I., Hayes, C., Hill, D. L. G., Leach, M. O., Hawkes, D. J. "Nonrigid registration using free-form deformations: application to breast MR images". *IEEE Trans Med Imag* 18 (8), 712–721, 1999.

[Rühaak et al. 2011] Rühaak, J., Heldmann, S., Fischer, B., "Improving Lung Registration by Incorporating Anatomical Knowledge: A Variational Approach". In: Beichel, R., de Bruijne, M., van Ginneken, B., Kabus, S., Kiraly, A., Kuhnigk, J. M., McClelland, J. R., Mori, K., van Rikxoort, E. M., Rit, S. (Eds.), Fourth International Workshop on Pulmonary Image Analysis, MICCAI 2011. pp. 147–156, 2011.

[Rühaak et al. 2013] Rühaak, J., Heldmann, S., Kipshagen, T., Fischer, B., "Highly accurate fast lung CT registration". In: Ourselin, S., Haynor, D. R. (Eds.), Proc SPIE. p. 86690Y, 2013.

[Samson et al. 1999] Samson, C., Blanc-Féraud, L., Zerubia, J., Aubert, G., "A Level Set Model for Image Classification". In: Nielsen, M., Johansen, P., Olsen, O. F., Weickert, J. (Eds.), Scale-Space Theories in Computer Vision: Second International Conference, Scale-Space '99. LNCS 1682. pp. 306–317, 1999.

[Sarrut 2006] Sarrut, D. "Deformable Registration for Image-Guided Radiation Therapy". *Z Med Phys*, 1–38, 2006.

[Sarrut et al. 2007] Sarrut, D., Delhay, S., Villard, P. "A comparison framework for breathing motion estimation methods from 4-D imaging". *IEEE Trans Med Imag* 26 (12), 1636–1648, 2007.

[Scatarige et al. 2003] Scatarige, J. C., Diette, G. B., Haponik, E. F., Merriman, B., Fishman, E. K. "Utility of High-Resolution CT for Management of Diffuse Lung Disease". *Acad Radiol* 10 (2), 167–175, 2003.

[Schmidt-Richberg et al. 2008] Schmidt-Richberg, A., Ehrhardt, J., Handels, H., "Variationeller Ansatz für eine integrierte Segmentierung und nicht-lineare Registrierung". In: Tolxdorff, T., Braun, J., Deserno, T. M., Horsch, A., Handels, H., Meinzer, H.-P. (Eds.), Bildverarbeitung für die Medizin. pp. 26–30, 2008.

[Schmidt-Richberg et al. 2009a] Schmidt-Richberg, A., Ehrhardt, J., Werner, R., Handels, H., "Evaluation and Comparison of Force Terms for the Estimation of Lung Motion by Non-linear Registration of 4D-CT Image Data". In: Dössel, O., Schlegel, W.

(Eds.), World Congress on Medical Physics and Biomedical Engineering. IFMBE Proceedings Volume 25/4. pp. 2128–2131, 2009.

[Schmidt-Richberg et al. 2009b] Schmidt-Richberg, A., Ehrhardt, J., Werner, R., Handels, H., "Slipping Objects in Image Registration: Improved Motion Field Estimation with Direction-Dependent Regularization". In: Yang, G.-Z., Hawkes, D. J., Rueckert, D., Noble, J. A., Taylor, C. (Eds.), Med Image Comput Comput Assist Interv. LNCS 5761. pp. 755–762, 2009.

[Schmidt-Richberg et al. 2010a] Schmidt-Richberg, A., Ehrhardt, J., Werner, R., Handels, H., "Diffeomorphic Diffusion Registration of Lung CT Images". In: van Ginneken, B., Murphy, K., Heimann, T., Pekar, V., Deng, X. (Eds.), Medical Image Analysis for the Clinic: A Grand Challenge, MICCAI 2010. pp. 55–62, 2010.

[Schmidt-Richberg et al. 2010b] Schmidt-Richberg, A., Ehrhardt, J., Werner, R., Handels, H., "Direction-Dependent Regularization for Improved Estimation of Liver and Lung Motion in 4D Image Data". In: Dawant, B. M., Haynor, D. R. (Eds.), Proc SPIE. p. 76232Y, 2010.

[Schmidt-Richberg et al. 2012a] Schmidt-Richberg, A., Ehrhardt, J., Werner, R., Handels, H., "Fast Explicit Diffusion for Registration with Direction-Dependent Regularization". In: Dawant, B. M., Christensen, G. E., Fitzpatrick, J. M., Rueckert, D. (Eds.), Biomedical Image Registration. LNCS 7359. pp. 220–228, 2012.

[Schmidt-Richberg et al. 2012b] Schmidt-Richberg, A., Ehrhardt, J., Werner, R., Handels, H., "Lung Registration with Improved Fissure Alignment by Integration of Pulmonary Lobe Segmentation". In: Ayache, N., Delingette, H., Golland, P., Mori, K. (Eds.), Med Image Comput Comput Assist Interv. LNCS 7511. pp. 74–81, 2012.

[Schmidt-Richberg et al. 2012c] Schmidt-Richberg, A., Ehrhardt, J., Werner, R., Wilms, M., Handels, H., "Evaluation of Algorithms for Lung Fissure Segmentation in CT Images". In: Tolxdorff, T., Deserno, T. M., Handels, H., Meinzer, H.-P. (Eds.), Bildverarbeitung für die Medizin. pp. 201–206, 2012.

[Schmidt-Richberg et al. 2012d] Schmidt-Richberg, A., Ehrhardt, J., Wilms, M., Werner, R., Handels, H., "Pulmonary Lobe Segmentation With Level Sets". In: Haynor, D. R., Ourselin, S. (Eds.), Proc SPIE. p. 83142V, 2012.

[Schmidt-Richberg et al. 2009c] Schmidt-Richberg, A., Handels, H., Ehrhardt, J. "Integrated segmentation and non-linear registration for organ segmentation and motion field estimation in 4D CT data". *Methods Inf Med* 48 (4), 344–349, 2009.

[Schmidt-Richberg et al. 2011] Schmidt-Richberg, A., Werner, R., Ehrhardt, J., Wolf, J.-C., Handels, H., "Landmark-driven parameter optimization for non-linear image registration". In: Dawant, B. M., Haynor, D. R. (Eds.), Proc SPIE. p. 79620T, 2011.

[Schmidt-Richberg et al. 2012e] Schmidt-Richberg, A., Werner, R., Handels, H., Ehrhardt, J. "Estimation of Slipping Organ Motion by Registration with Direction-Dependent Regularization". *Med Image Anal* 16 (1), 150–159, 2012.

[Seiler et al. 2012] Seiler, C., Pennec, X., Reyes, M., "Simultaneous Multiscale Polyaffine Registration by Incorporating Deformation Statistics". In: Ayache, N., Delingette, H., Golland, P., Mori, K. (Eds.), Med Image Comput Comput Assist Interv. LNCS 7511. pp. 130–137, 2012.

[Sheng and Cai 2008] Sheng, K., Cai, J. "TH-C-AUD C-01: Lung Mechanical Modeling Based On the 3He MR Tagging and Lobar Segmentation". *Med Phys* 35 (6), 2972, 2008.

[Shi et al. 2012] Shi, W., Zhuang, X., Pizarro, L., Bai, W., Wang, H., Tung, K.-P., Edwards, P., Rueckert, D., "Registration Using Sparse Free-Form Deformations". In: Ayache, N., Delingette, H., Golland, P., Mori, K. (Eds.), Med Image Comput Comput Assist Interv. LNCS 7511. pp. 659–666, 2012.

[Shimizu et al. 2001] Shimizu, S., Shirato, H., Ogura, S., Akita-Dosaka, H., Kitamura, K., Nishioka, T., Kagei, K., Nishimura, M., Miyasaka, K. "Detection of lung tumor movement in real-time tumor-tracking radiotherapy". *Int J Radiat Oncol Biol Phys* 51 (2), 304–310, 2001.

[Sluimer et al. 2006] Sluimer, I., Schilham, A. M. R., Prokop, M., van Ginneken, B. "Computer Analysis of Computed Tomography Scans of the Lung: A Survey". *IEEE Trans Med Imag* 25 (4), 385–405, 2006.

[Song et al. 2010] Song, G., Tustison, N. J., Avants, B. B., Gee, J. C., "Lung CT Image Registration Using Diffeomorphic Transformation Models". In: van Ginneken, B., Murphy, K., Heimann, T., Pekar, V., Deng, X. (Eds.), Medical Image Analysis for the Clinic: A Grand Challenge, MICCAI 2010. pp. 23–32, 2010.

[Song et al. 2006] Song, T., Lee, V. S., Rusinek, H., Wong, S., Laine, A. F., "Integrated Four Dimensional Registration and Segmentation of Dynamic Renal MR Images". In: Larsen, R., Nielsen, M., Sporring, J. (Eds.), Med Image Comput Comput Assist Interv. LNCS 4191. pp. 758–765, 2006.

[Sotiras et al. 2012] Sotiras, A., Davatazikos, C., Paragios, N., "Deformable Medical Image Registration: A Survey". Tech. Rep. 7919, INRIA, 2012.

[Staring et al. 2010] Staring, M., Klein, S., Reiber, J. H. C., Niessen, W. J., Stoel, B. C., "Pulmonary Image Registration with elastix using a Standard Intensity-Based Algorithm". In: van Ginneken, B., Murphy, K., Heimann, T., Pekar, V., Deng, X. (Eds.), Medical Image Analysis for the Clinic: A Grand Challenge, MICCAI 2010. pp. 73–79, 2010.

[Staring et al. 2009] Staring, M., Pluim, J. P. W., de Hoop, B. J., Klein, S., van Ginneken, B., Gietema, H. A., Nossent, G., Schaefer-Prokop, C., van de Vorst, S., Prokop, M. "Image subtraction facilitates assessment of volume and density change in ground-glass opacities in chest CT". *Invest Radiol* 44 (2), 61–66, 2009.

[Studholme et al. 1999] Studholme, C., Hill, D. L. G., Hawkes, D. J. "An overlap invariant entropy measure of 3D medical image alignment". *Pattern Recognit* 32 (1), 71–86, 1999.

[Sun et al. 2008] Sun, D., Roth, S., Lewis, J. P., Black, M. J., "Learning Optical Flow". In: Forsyth, D., Torr, P., Zisserman, A. (Eds.), Europ Conf Comp Vis. pp. 83–97, 2008.

[Thirion 1995] Thirion, J.-P., "Fast Non-Rigid Matching of 3D Medical Images". Tech. Rep. 2547, INRIA, France, 1995.

[Thirion 1998] Thirion, J.-P. "Image matching as a diffusion process: an analogy with Maxwell's demons". *Med Image Anal* 2 (3), 243–260, 1998.

[Trouvé 1998] Trouvé, A. "Diffeomorphisms Groups and Pattern Matching in Image Analysis". *Int J Comput Vis* 28 (3), 213–221, 1998.

[Tustison et al. 2011] Tustison, N. J., Cook, T. S., Song, G., Gee, J. C. "Pulmonary kinematics from image data: a review". *Acad Radiol* 18 (4), 402–417, 2011.

[Ukil and Reinhardt 2009] Ukil, S., Reinhardt, J. M. "Anatomy-Guided Lung Lobe Segmentation in X-Ray CT Images". *IEEE Trans Med Imag* 28 (2), 202–214, 2009.

[Unal and Slabaugh 2005] Unal, G., Slabaugh, G., "Coupled PDEs for non-rigid registration and segmentation". In: Proc IEEE Comput Soc Conf Comput Vis Pattern Recognit. pp. 168–175, 2005.

[van Rikxoort et al. 2009] van Rikxoort, E. M., de Hoop, B. J., Viergever, M. A., Prokop, M., van Ginneken, B. "Automatic lung segmentation from thoracic computed tomography scans using a hybrid approach with error detection". *Med Phys* 36 (7), 2934–2947, 2009.

[van Rikxoort et al. 2010] van Rikxoort, E. M., Prokop, M., de Hoop, B. J., Viergever, M. A., Pluim, J. P. W., van Ginneken, B. "Automatic Segmentation of Pulmonary Lobes Robust against Incomplete Fissures". *IEEE Trans Med Imag* 29 (6), 1286–1296, 2010.

[van Rikxoort et al. 2008] van Rikxoort, E. M., van Ginneken, B., Klik, M., Prokop, M. "Supervised Enhancement Filters: Application to Fissure Detection in Chest CT Scans". *IEEE Trans Med Imag* 27 (1), 1–10, 2008.

[Vandemeulebroucke et al. 2012] Vandemeulebroucke, J., Bernard, O., Rit, S., Kybic, J., Clarysse, P., Sarrut, D. "Automated segmentation of a motion mask to preserve sliding motion in deformable registration of thoracic CT". *Med Phys* 39 (2), 1006–1015, 2012.

[Vandemeulebroucke et al. 2007] Vandemeulebroucke, J., Sarrut, D., Clarysse, P., "The POPI-model, a point-validated pixel-based breathing thorax model". In: Proc ICCR, 2007.

[Vasilescu and Terzopoulos 1992] Vasilescu, M., Terzopoulos, D., "Adaptive Meshes and Shells: Irregular Triangulation, Discontinuities, and Hierarchical Subdivision". In: Proc IEEE Comput Soc Conf Comput Vis Pattern Recognit. pp. 829–832, 1992.

[Vercauteren et al. 2009] Vercauteren, T., Pennec, X., Perchant, A. "Diffeomorphic demons: Efficient non-parametric image registration". *NeuroImage* 45, S61–S72, 2009.

[Vercauteren et al. 2007] Vercauteren, T., Pennec, X., Perchant, A., Ayache, N., "Non-parametric Diffeomorphic Image Registration with the Demons Algorithm". In: Ayache, N., Ourselin, S., Maeder, A. (Eds.), Med Image Comput Comput Assist Interv. LNCS 4792. pp. 319–326, 2007.

[Viola and Wells 1995] Viola, P., Wells, III, W. M., "Alignment by maximization of mutual information". In: Proc IEEE Int Conf Comput Vis. pp. 16–23, 1995.

[von Siebenthal et al. 2007] von Siebenthal, M., Székely, G., Gamper, U., Boesiger, P. "4D MR imaging of respiratory organ motion and its variability". *Phys Med Biol* 52 (6), 1547–1564, 2007.

[Wang et al. 2005] Wang, H., Dong, L., O'Daniel, J., Mohan, R., Garden, A. S., Ang, K. K., Kuban, D. A., Bonnen, M., Chang, J. Y., Cheung, R. "Validation of an accelerated 'demons' algorithm for deformable image registration in radiation therapy". *Phys Med Biol* 50 (12), 2887–2905, 2005.

[Wang et al. 2006] Wang, J., Betke, M., Ko, J. P. "Pulmonary fissure segmentation on CT". *Med Image Anal* 10 (4), 530–547, 2006.

[Weickert et al. 1998] Weickert, J., Romeny, B. M. t. H., Viergever, M. A. "Efficient and Reliable Schemes for Nonlinear Diffusion Filtering". *IEEE Trans Image Process* 7 (3), 398–410, 1998.

[Werner 2012] Werner, R., "Bewegungsfeldschätzung und Dosisakkumulation anhand von 4D-Bilddaten für die Strahlentherapie atmungsbewegter Tumoren". Ph.D. thesis, University of Lübeck, 2012.

[Werner et al. 2009a] Werner, R., Ehrhardt, J., Schmidt, R., Handels, H. "Patient-specific finite element modeling of respiratory lung motion using 4D CT image data". *Med Phys* 36 (5), 1500–1511, 2009.

[Werner et al. 2012a] Werner, R., Ehrhardt, J., Schmidt-Richberg, A., Albers, D., Frenzel, T., Petersen, C., Cremers, F., Handels, H. "Towards Accurate Dose Accumulation for Step-&-Shoot IMRT: Impact of Weighting Schemes and Temporal Image Resolution on the Estimation of Dosimetric Motion Effects". *Z Med Phys* 22 (2), 109–122, 2012.

[Werner et al. 2009b] Werner, R., Ehrhardt, J., Schmidt-Richberg, A., Handels, H., "Validation and comparison of a biophysical modeling approach and non-linear registration for estimation of lung motion fields in thoracic 4D CT data". In: Pluim, J. P. W., Dawant, B. M. (Eds.), Proc SPIE. p. 72590U, 2009.

[Werner et al. 2012b] Werner, R., Ehrhardt, J., Schmidt-Richberg, A., Handels, H., "Model-based risk assessment for motion effects in 3D radiotherapy of lung tumors". In: Holmes III, D. R., Wong, K. H. (Eds.), Proc SPIE. p. 83160C, 2012.

[Whitaker 1998] Whitaker, R. T. "A Level-Set Approach to 3D Reconstruction from Range Data". *Int J Comput Vis* 29 (3), 203–231, 1998.

[Wiemker et al. 2005] Wiemker, R., Bülow, T., Blaffert, T., "Unsupervised extraction of the pulmonary interlobar fissures from high resolution thoracic CT data". In: Lemke, H. U., Inamura, K., Doi, K., Vannier, M. W., Farman, A. G. (Eds.), Proc CARS. pp. 1121–1126, 2005.

[Wilms et al. 2012] Wilms, M., Ehrhardt, J., Handels, H., "A 4D Statistical Shape Model for Automated Segmentation of Lungs with Large Tumors". In: Ayache, N., Delingette, H., Golland, P., Mori, K. (Eds.), Med Image Comput Comput Assist Interv. LNCS 7511. pp. 347–354, 2012.

[Witkin 1983] Witkin, A., "Scale-space filtering". In: Proc 8th Int Joint Conf Art Intel. pp. 1019–1022, 1983.

[Wolz et al. 2010] Wolz, R., Aljabar, P., Hajnal, J. V., Hammers, A., Rueckert, D., Alzheimer's Disease Neuroimaging Initiative. "LEAP: learning embeddings for atlas propagation". *NeuroImage* 49 (2), 1316–1325, 2010.

[Wu et al. 2008] Wu, Z., Rietzel, E., Boldea, V., Sarrut, D., Sharp, G. C. "Evaluation of deformable registration of patient lung 4DCT with subanatomical region segmentations". *Med Phys* 35 (2), 775, 2008.

[Wyatt and Noble 2003] Wyatt, P. P., Noble, J. A. "MAP MRF joint segmentation and registration of medical images". *Med Image Anal* 7 (4), 539–552, 2003.

[Xie et al. 2009] Xie, Y., Chao, M., Xing, L. "Tissue Feature-Based and Segmented Deformable Image Registration for Improved Modeling of Shear Movement of Lungs". *Int J Radiat Oncol Biol Phys* 74 (4), 1256–1265, 2009.

[Yan et al. 1999] Yan, D., Jaffray, D. A., Wong, J. W. "A model to accumulate fractionated dose in a deforming organ". *Int J Radiat Oncol Biol Phys* 44 (3), 665–675, 1999.

[Yang et al. 2008] Yang, D., Lu, W., Low, D. A., Deasy, J. O., Hope, A. J., El Naqa, I. "4D-CT motion estimation using deformable image registration and 5D respiratory motion modeling". *Med Phys* 35 (10), 4577–4590, 2008.

[Yezzi et al. 2003] Yezzi, A., Zöllei, L., Kapur, T. "A variational framework for integrating segmentation and registration through active contours". *Med Image Anal* 7 (2), 171–185, 2003.

[Yin et al. 2009] Yin, Y., Hoffman, E. A., Lin, C.-L. "Mass preserving nonrigid registration of CT lung images using cubic B-spline". *Med Phys* 36 (9), 4213–4222, 2009.

[Yin et al. 2010] Yin, Y., Hoffman, E. A., Lin, C.-L., "Lung Lobar Slippage Assessed with the Aid of Image Registration". In: Jiang, T., Navab, N., Pluim, J. P. W., Viergever, M. A. (Eds.), Med Image Comput Comput Assist Interv. LNCS 6362. pp. 578–585, 2010.

[Younes et al. 2009] Younes, L., Arrate, F., Miller, M. I. "Evolutions equations in computational anatomy". *NeuroImage* 45 (1), S40–S50, 2009.

[Young and Levy 2005] Young, Y.-N., Levy, D. "Registration-based morphing of active contours for segmentation of CT scans". *Math Biosci Eng* 2 (1), 79–96, 2005.

[Zhang et al. 2006] Zhang, L., Hoffman, E. A., Reinhardt, J. M. "Atlas-Driven Lung Lobe Segmentation in Volumetric X-Ray CT Images". *IEEE Trans Med Imag* 25 (1), 1–16, 2006.

[Zhao et al. 1996] Zhao, H.-K., Chan, T. F., Merriman, B., Osher, S. "A variational level set approach to multiphase motion". *J Comp Phys* 127, 179–195, 1996.

[Zheng et al. 2007] Zheng, Y., Steiner, K., Bauer, T., Yu, J., Shen, D., Kambhamettu, C., "Lung Nodule Growth Analysis from 3D CT Data with a Coupled Segmentation and Registration Framework". In: Proc IEEE Int Conf Comput Vis. pp. 1–8, 2007.

[Zimmer et al. 2009] Zimmer, H., Bruhn, A., Weickert, J., Valgaerts, L., "Complementary Optic Flow". In: Cremers, D., Boykov, Y., Blake, A., Schmidt, F. R. (Eds.), Proc EMMCVPR. LNCS 5681. pp. 207–220, 2009.

[Zitova and Flusser 2003] Zitova, B., Flusser, J. "Image registration methods: a survey". *Image Vis Comput* 21 (11), 977–1000, 2003.

Aktuelle Forschung Medizintechnik

Herausgeber:

Prof. Dr. Thorsten M. Buzug

Institut für Medizintechnik, Universität zu Lübeck

Themen
Werke aus folgenden Themengebieten werden gerne in die Reihe aufgenommen: Biomedizinische Mikro- und Nanosysteme, Elektromedizin, biomedizinische Mess- und Sensortechnik, Monitoring, Lasertechnik, Robotik, minimalinvasive Chirurgie, integrierte OP-Systeme, bildgebende Verfahren, digitale Bildverarbeitung und Visualisierung, Kommunikations- und Informationssysteme, Telemedizin, eHealth und wissensbasierte Systeme, Biosignalverarbeitung, Modellierung und Simulation, Biomechanik, aktive und passive Implantate, Tissue Engineering, Neuroprothetik, Dosimetrie, Strahlenschutz, Strahlentherapie.

Autorinnen und Autoren
Autoren der Reihe sind in der Regel junge Promovierte und Habilitierte, die exzellente Abschlussarbeiten verfasst haben.

Leserschaft
Die Reihe wendet sich einerseits an Studierende, Promovenden und Habilitanden aus den Bereichen Medizintechnik, Medizinische Ingenieurwissenschaft, Medizinische Physik, Medizinische Informatik oder ähnlicher Richtungen. Andererseits stellt die Reihe aktuelle Arbeiten aus einem sich schnell entwickelnden Feld dar, so dass auch Wissenschaftlerinnen und Wissenschaftler sowie Entwicklerinnen und Entwickler an Universitäten, in außeruniversitären Forschungseinrichtungen und der Industrie von den ausgewählten Arbeiten in innovativen Gebieten der Medizintechnik profitieren werden.

Begutachtungsprozess
Die Qualitätssicherung erfolgt in drei Schritten. Zunächst werden nur Arbeiten angenommen die mindestens magna cum laude bewertet sind. Im zweiten Schritt wird ein Mitglied des Editorial Boards die Annahme oder Ablehnung des Werkes empfehlen. Im letzten Schritt wird der Reihenherausgeber über die Annahme oder Ablehnung entscheiden sowie Änderungen in der Druckfassung empfehlen. Die Koordination übernimmt der Reihenherausgeber.

Kontakt
Prof. Dr. Thorsten M. Buzug
Institut für Medizintechnik
Universität zu Lübeck
Ratzeburger Allee 160
23538 Lübeck, Germany

Tel.: +49 (0) 451 / 500-5400
Fax: +49 (0) 451 / 500-5403
E-Mail: buzug@imt.uni-luebeck.de
Web: http://www.imt.uni-luebeck.de

Stand: Mai 2012. Änderungen vorbehalten.
Erhältlich im Buchhandel oder beim Verlag.

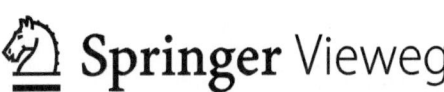

Abraham-Lincoln-Straße 46
D-65189 Wiesbaden
Tel. +49 (0)6221. 345 - 4301
www.springer-vieweg.de